Inhaled Delivery Systems for the Treatment of Asthma and COPD

Inhaled therapies form the cornerstone for treatment of patients with asthma and COPD. Evolving technology has resulted in availability of a wide range of devices for delivery of inhaled drugs. The four different delivery systems – pressurized metered-dose inhalers, slow mist inhalers, dry powder inhalers, and nebulizers – are unique in design and require distinct inhalational instructions for correct use. This book provides current information about inhalation devices, including their advantages and disadvantages, with guidance for optimal techniques of use. The book emphasizes appropriate selection of inhalation devices based on patient and health care professional factors, as well as device attributes that allow selection of the right medication in the right inhalation device at the right time for the right patient.

Key features:

- Addresses the objective of precision medicine – the right medication in the right inhaler device at the right time.

- Inputs by international thought leaders who have published widely on inhaled medications and/or inhaled delivery systems for clinicians, trainees, and respiratory therapists.

- Discusses the development of audio-based systems and smart inhalers for patient monitoring.

T0139074

Inhaled Delivery Systems for the Treatment of Asthma and COPD

Edited By

Donald A. Mahler, MD
Emeritus Professor of Medicine
Geisel School of Medicine at Dartmouth
Hanover, New Hampshire, USA

Director of Respiratory Services
Valley Regional Hospital
Claremont, New Hampshire, USA

Rajiv Dhand, MD
Professor and Wahid T. Hanna MD Endowed Chair
Department of Medicine
Associate Dean of Clinical Affairs
University of Tennessee Graduate School of Medicine
Knoxville, Tennessee, USA

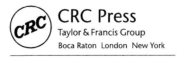

CRC Press
Taylor & Francis Group
Boca Raton London New York

CRC Press is an imprint of the
Taylor & Francis Group, an **informa** business

CRC Press
Boca Raton and London

First edition published 2023
by CRC Press
6000 Broken Sound Parkway NW, Suite 300, Boca Raton, FL 33487-2742

and by CRC Press
4 Park Square, Milton Park, Abingdon, Oxon, OX14 4RN

CRC Press is an imprint of Taylor & Francis Group, LLC

© 2023 selection and editorial matter, Donald A. Mahler and Rajiv Dhand; individual chapters, the contributors

Library of Congress Cataloging-in-Publication Data

Names: Mahler, Donald A., editor. | Dhand, Rajiv, editor.
Title: Inhaled delivery systems for the treatment of asthma and COPD / edited by Donald A. Mahler, Rajiv Dhand.
Description: First edition. | Boca Raton : CRC Press, 2023. | Includes bibliographical references and index.
Identifiers: LCCN 2023000038 (print) | LCCN 2023000039 (ebook) | ISBN 9781032215730 (paperback) | ISBN 9781032215747 (hardback) | ISBN 9781003269014 (ebook)
Subjects: MESH: Asthma--drug therapy | Pulmonary Disease, Chronic Obstructive--drug therapy | Administration, Inhalation | Respiratory Therapy--methods | Nebulizers and Vaporizers | Aerosols
Classification: LCC RC591 (print) | LCC RC591 (ebook) | NLM WF 648 | DDC 616.2/38061--dc23/eng/20230505
LC record available at https://lccn.loc.gov/2023000038
LC ebook record available at https://lccn.loc.gov/2023000039

ISBN: 978-1-032-21574-7 (hbk)
ISBN: 978-1-032-21573-0 (pbk)
ISBN: 978-1-003-26901-4 (ebk)

DOI: 10.1201/9781003269014

Typeset in Palatino
by KnowledgeWorks Global Ltd.

Table of Contents

Foreword

Inhalation is the preferred route of administration of nearly all medications for the treatment of asthma and COPD via various hand-held devices or nebulizer systems. While hand-held devices are commonly used because of their relative simplicity and convenience, technical challenges to their correct use are frequently not met, resulting in ineffective delivery of these medications to the lungs, thus undermining their clinical benefit. Nebulizer systems for medication delivery, while less convenient than hand-held devices, are most often used in the hospital and emergency room settings and serve as valuable alternatives to hand-held devices in outpatients who are unable to master the technical challenges to their effective use. Asthma and COPD affect hundreds of millions of people worldwide, and COPD is the third leading cause of death globally, underscoring the vital importance of effective delivery of inhaled medications.

Drs. Donald A. Mahler and Rajiv Dhand, two widely recognized and highly respected authorities on inhaled delivery systems with whom I have had the distinct privilege to serve in various committees and conferences related to aerosol therapy, have assembled an international group of distinguished experts to contribute to their book a total of 14 chapters covering a wide range of key topics relevant to inhaled delivery systems for treating asthma and COPD, in addition to other respiratory diseases (cystic fibrosis, bronchiectasis, and pulmonary hypertension) responsive to a variety of medications deliverable by the inhaled route.

Their book is an up-to-date and comprehensive review of the mechanics and technical aspects of differing inhaled delivery systems, the requirements for their optimal use by both adult and pediatric patients, their relative advantages and disadvantages depending on host characteristics, their use in different clinical settings and for the treatment of different respiratory disorders, the ongoing development of "smart" inhalers utilizing advanced digital technology to optimize delivery technique, patient adherence, and the physician-patient relationship, and practical issues regarding cost and patient access in the current regulatory environment. As such, the book serves as a uniquely valuable resource for a variety of health care professionals, as well as inhalational device manufacturers.

Donald P. Tashkin, MD, FCCP, ATSF
Distinguished Emeritus Professor of Medicine
Division of Pulmonary and Critical Care Medicine, Clinical Immunology & Allergy
David Geffen School of Medicine at UCLA

About the Editors

Donald A. Mahler (MD, FCCP) is Emeritus Professor of Medicine at Geisel School of Medicine at Dartmouth in Hanover, New Hampshire. He currently works as a pulmonary physician at Valley Regional Hospital in Claremont, New Hampshire, where he is Director of Respiratory Services.

His research interests include the evaluation/treatment of dyspnea and clinical outcomes in COPD. Under the mentorship of the late Alvin Feinstein, MD, Dr. Mahler developed and established the psychometric properties of the interviewer-administered baseline and transition dyspnea indexes (BDI/TDI), which have been translated into over 80 languages. The BDI/TDI have been used as an outcome measure in phase 3 clinical trials involving medications approved by the Food and Drug Administration and/or the European Medicines Agency for treatment of patients with COPD. These include Serevent®, Spriva®, Advair®, Brovana®, Tudorza®, Daliresp®, Arcapta®, Ultibro®, Anoro®, Striverdi®, Stiolto®, Utibron®, and Yupelri®.

In collaboration with the late John C. Baird, PhD, the interviewer administered BDI/TDI were converted into self-administered and computerized (SAC) versions, enabling patients to provide a direct rating of breathlessness during daily activities. The SAC versions have been translated into 12 languages and have been included as an outcome measure in phase 3 and 4 clinical trials evaluating therapies for patients with interstitial lung disease and COPD.

Dr. Mahler has authored/co-authored over 180 original research articles and over 100 editorials, book chapters, and non-peer-reviewed articles. In addition, he has written/edited four books on dyspnea.

In June 2014, he created the website, https://www.donaldmahler.com, with the vision "to positively affect the daily lives of those with COPD and their families." In February 2015, Dr. Mahler authored *COPD: Answers to Your Questions* (Two Harbors Press) to address the common questions posed by those with COPD, family members, and their caregivers. In January 2022, he wrote *COPD: Answers to Your Most Pressing Questions about Chronic Obstructive Pulmonary Disease* (Johns Hopkins University Press).

Dr. Rajiv Dhand (MD, FCCP, FACP, FAARC, FRSM, ATSF) serves as Professor of Medicine with tenure, the Wahid T. Hanna MD Endowed Chair of the Department of Medicine, Service Chief of the Medical Service and Associate Dean of Clinical Affairs at the University of Tennessee, Graduate School of Medicine in Knoxville, TN. Previously, he served as Division Director of Pulmonary, Critical Care, and Environmental Medicine at the University of Missouri. He is a Past President of the International Society of Aerosols in Medicine (ISAM).

Dr. Dhand is a skilled pulmonologist who is internationally recognized for his work on inhaled therapies. He helped to establish the scientific basis for the use of metered-dose inhalers in mechanically ventilated patients. He was an invited member of several Task Forces that developed Guidelines on Aerosolization of Medication that were published in *CHEST*, *European Respiratory Journal*, and *Journal of Aerosol Medicine and Pulmonary Drug Delivery*.

Dr. Dhand served as a principal investigator on many clinical trials over the past 20 years, principally related to bronchodilator therapy in patients with chronic obstructive pulmonary disease (COPD). His experience includes studies in experimental, translational, and clinical research and he is the recipient of several research grants during his career.

Dr. Dhand has been awarded Fellowships of the American College of Physicians, American College of Chest Physicians, American Thoracic Society, Royal Society of Medicine, American Association of Respiratory Care, and International Society of Aerosols in Medicine. He is Editor-in-Chief of the *ISAM Textbook of Aerosol Medicine*. Dr. Dhand has held multiple editorial appointments including *CHEST, Journal of Aerosol Medicine and Pulmonary Drug Delivery, Respiratory Care,* and *International Journal of COPD*. He is the Respiratory Section editor for *Advances in Therapy* and US Editor-in-Chief of *Pulmonary Therapy* Journal. He has published over 170 articles in peer-reviewed journals and has lectured at a host of national and international venues. He remains actively engaged in clinical practice as well as teaching and training medical students, internal medicine residents, and pulmonary/critical care medicine fellows.

Contributors

Israel Amirav
Professor
Pediatric Pulmonology Unit
Dana-Dwek Children's Hospital
Tel Aviv Medical Center
Tel Aviv University
Tel Aviv, Israel

Isaac N. Biney
Assistant Professor
Division of Pulmonary and Critical
Care Medicine
Graduate School of Medicine
Knoxville, Tennessee

Rajiv Dhand
Professor of Medicine
Wahid T. Hanna MD Endowed
Chair of Medicine
Associate Dean of Clinical Affairs
Graduate School of Medicine
Knoxville, Tennessee

Myrna B. Dolovich
Professor of Medicine (Part-time)
McMaster University
Head, Firestone Research Aerosol Lab
Affiliate, Research Institute of St Joes
St Joseph's Hospital, Hamilton
Ontario, Canada

Alexander G. Duarte
Professor
Pulmonary, Critical Care and Sleep
Medicine
University of Texas Medical Branch
Galveston, Texas

Mahmoud M. Ibrahim
Pulmonary, Critical Care and Sleep
Medicine
University of Texas Medical Branch
Galveston, Texas

Jie Li
Department of Cardiopulmonary
Sciences
Division of Respiratory Care
Rush University
Chicago, Illinois

Bruce K. Rubin
Distinguished Professor of Pediatrics
and Biomedical Engineering
Virginia Eminent Scholar in
Pediatrics
Virginia Commonwealth University
School of Medicine
Richmond, Virginia

Francisco J. Soto
Associate Professor of Medicine
Director, Pulmonary Vascular
Disease
Division of Pulmonary and Critical
Care Medicine
Graduate School of Medicine
Knoxville, Tennessee

Paul D. Terry
Professor
Department of Medicine
Graduate School of Medicine
Knoxville, Tennessee

Introduction

Donald A. Mahler and Rajiv Dhand

Inhaled therapies are the cornerstone of treatment for individuals with asthma and COPD. To be effective, patients need to inhale the medication deep into the lower respiratory tract to activate receptors that dilate airways or reduce airway inflammation. Although both the specific molecule(s) and the delivery system are important for effective therapy, the major focus by professional respiratory organizations and pharmaceutical companies has been on development and promotion of specific molecule(s). Unfortunately, there has been limited guidance on the selection of the most appropriate inhaled delivery system for the individual patient. The four different delivery systems – pressurized metered-dose inhalers, slow mist inhalers, dry powder inhalers, and nebulizers – are unique in design and require distinct inhalational instructions for correct use by patients.

The purpose of writing this book is to address an important, but neglected topic: What should health care professionals consider when selecting an inhaled delivery system for an individual with asthma or COPD? A new resource is needed for several reasons:

1. Increased awareness of the high prevalence of incorrect inhalational technique among users.

2. The unique features of the four different inhaled delivery systems.

3. Emerging evidence that various patient factors (e.g., age, sex, cognitive function, manual dexterity, and peak inspiratory flow) affect optimal use of the inhaled delivery system.

4. The development of audio-based and digital systems for monitoring correct inhaler technique.

This book addresses the objective of precision medicine – selecting the right medication *in the right inhalation device* at the right time. The 14 chapters provide guidance for health care professionals to match an inhaled delivery system with the individual patient who has asthma and/or COPD. Moreover, this information enhances understanding about the appropriate use and care of inhaled delivery systems. Finally, we hope that the contents of the book provide a springboard for addressing new research questions.

1 Principles of Inhaled Therapy

Omar S. Usmani and Federico Lavorini

CONTENTS

INTRODUCTION

Delivering drugs using the inhalation route to the lungs is the foundation of the everyday clinical management of patients with airway diseases (1–3). The inhaled route, as opposed to systemic drug administration, allows key therapeutic benefits. Targeting the drugs to the site of action in the lungs achieves a quicker onset of action, a reduction in the dose of drug used, and an improved therapeutic ratio (efficacy to adverse event ratio). The global pandemic has seen a seismic need for us to understand aerosol science, for example, infectious aerosols and therapeutic aerosols (4). In this chapter we discuss the physiochemical factors that control the transport, delivery, and deposition of inhaled drug within the lungs.

MECHANISMS OF DRUG DEPOSITION IN THE LUNGS

Inhaled drug deposition is an active process that requires the inspired therapeutic particles to be maximally retained within the airways of the lungs and minimize loss of drug in the exhaled air (5, 6). The chief mechanisms that control inhaled medical aerosol deposition within the airways are inertial impaction, sedimentation, and diffusion (Figure 1.1) (7, 8).

These physical mechanisms act concurrently on the inhaled drug particles as they follow the airstream on their trajectory within the respiratory tract and collectively contribute to the deposition of aerosolized drug within the lungs. The relative proportions and extent to which each mechanism contributes and predominates are dependent on the physicochemical properties of the drug particle, the pathology and geometry of the local airways, the airstream parameters, and the inhalation maneuver and pattern of breathing of the patient

Inertial Impaction

Inertial impaction of inhaled drug particles occurs when the forward momentum of an individual drug particle causes it to maintain its original path and direction of flow in the airstream leading it to impact on the surrounding airway wall, in a region of the respiratory tract where there is a change in the bulk direction of the airstream. Inertial impaction predominantly occurs with inhaled drug particles at airway bifurcations in larger branches of the airways

DOI: 10.1201/9781003269014-1

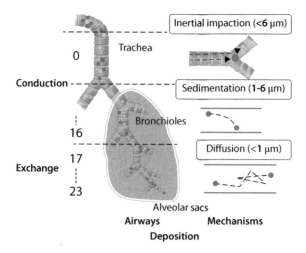

Figure 1.1 Mechanisms of aerosol deposition in the airways.

in the respiratory tract where the velocities of airflow are high and where rapid and fast changes occur in the path and direction of the airstream (Figure 1.1).

Impaction of inhaled drug particles within the lungs is beneficial. However, inertial impaction is also the prime determinant of drug depositing within the oropharynx that can lead to unwanted local adverse effects and through oral bioavailability, depending upon the pharmacokinetic behavior and metabolism of the drug systemic adverse effects. The ballistic high-velocity nature of the aerosol spray emitted from inhaler devices, such as some pressurized metered-dose inhalers (pMDIs), or inhaled with intense inspiratory force and flows by the patients, as is needed with some dry powder inhalers (DPIs), can lead to significant proportions of the emitted drug particles impacting within the oropharynx and minimal amounts, in some cases less than 20%, reaching the lungs (9–11).

Inhaler devices have evolved to slow down the emitted aerosol spray and plume velocity, such as newer pMDIs with refined drug formulations (12), the slow mist inhaler (SMI) (13), and DPIs requiring gentler inhalation flows (14) that can decrease oropharyngeal impaction. In clinical practice, valve-holding chambers (VHCs) and spacers are sometimes used and attached to pMDIs that allow an extension to the inhaler mouthpiece, and by increasing the distance the aerosol spray has to travel, VHCs slow down the velocity of the aerosol spray, which has a two-fold effect (15, 16). First, VHCs allow time for the aerosol propellant to evaporate and this results in smaller drug particles that have greater potential to reach the lower respiratory tract compared to large inhaled drug particles (17), and secondly the ballistic impact of the aerosolized drug within the oropharyngeal cavity is reduced (15). The slow mist inhaler emits an aerosol spray that is slow and steady with a longer duration compared to pMDIs containing a greater fraction of fine particles (18, 19). Inertial impaction and gravitational sedimentation are the main mechanisms that influence the deposition of large, fast-moving inhaled particles of drug between 1μm and 10μm.

Gravitational Sedimentation

Gravitational sedimentation of inhaled drug particles within the lungs occurs under the action of gravity and causes deposition within the airways when the gravitational force acting on a drug particle overcomes the total force of air resistance. Sedimentation occurs where the velocity of the airstream is low allowing the available time for the inhaled drug particles to settle within the airway (residence time), being most efficient in the branching small airways where the distance to deposit on the airway walls is smaller compared to the larger airways (Figure 1.1). The breath-hold pause instruction often given to patients after inhalation of the aerosol enhances the action of sedimentation on inhaled drug particles in achieving greater airway deposition (20).

Diffusion

Diffusion is the random collision of gas molecules of air present in the airways with very small particles, in this case inhaled drug particles, which displaces and pushes the aerosolized drug particles about within the airways, in an irregular and erratic manner (5). As a consequence of diffusion, a drug particle in stationary air continues to move around in a random manner, even in the absence of gravity, and this can lead the inhaled drug particles to contact and deposit on the surrounding airway wall. Diffusion predominantly occurs in the distal small airways and alveoli, where airflow velocities are at their lowest, the residence time within the airways is long, and the distance an inhaled particle has to travel before hitting the airway wall is short (Figure 1.1). Diffusion is the main deposition determinant of slow-moving, small submicron (<1 μm) particles.

FACTORS AFFECTING DEPOSITION

Many factors can influence the deposition of inhaled aerosolized drug particles within the airways and they can generally be divided into aerosol characteristics and patient variables (Table 1.1).

Table 1.1: Factors Affecting Airways Deposition of Inhaled Medical Aerosols

Aerosol Factors	Patient Factors
Drug particle characteristics:	Inhalation maneuver:
<ul><li>particle density</li><li>particle electrostatics</li><li>particle shape</li><li>particle size and fraction</li></ul>	<ul><li>breathing frequency</li><li>breath-hold pause</li><li>chin lift</li><li>degree of lung inflation</li><li>exhalation to end tidal breath before inhalation</li><li>inhaled aerosol volume</li><li>inspiratory flow</li><li>nose vs. mouth breathing</li></ul>
Drug formulation:	Airway features:
<ul><li>hygroscopicity</li><li>surfactant</li><li>molecule charge</li></ul>	<ul><li>adult vs. pediatric</li><li>airways disease type</li><li>diameter and obstruction</li><li>severity of disease</li></ul>
Aerosol generation system:	Healthcare features:
<ul><li>inhaler device type</li><li>maintenance of device</li></ul>	<ul><li>competency of healthcare to teach, train and instruct patient</li><li>inhaler regimen</li><li>patient adherence</li><li>patient technique</li></ul>

Aerosol Properties

Of the physicochemical aerosol properties, drug particle size, or mass median aerodynamic diameter (MMAD) for therapeutic aerosols, is the most significant factor that determines the overall amount of inhaled drug particles depositing within the lungs and also the distribution of aerosolized drug within the airway regions. The branching airway system of the respiratory tract acts primarily as a defense mechanism analogous to a series of filters sequentially removing harmful airborne particulate matter from the inspired airstream. Inhaled drug particles therefore need to overcome the barriers to achieve effective drug deposition. Generally, inhaled particles >100 microns in size are usually trapped in the upper airway nasal cavity, where those >10 micron typically deposit in the oropharyngeal region, and particles between 2 and 6 microns deposit in the conducting airways. Extra fine inhaled drug particles, defined as those less than 2.1 microns (21), have the best potential to reach the small airways and distal lung region.

It is clear that modulating the particle size of inhaled drug can optimize drug delivery to the lungs and the clinical benefit experienced by the patients in terms of impact on their disease (22–24). Indeed, this will depend upon the drug class and pharmacological action of the drug and also the lung region it is thought best to target the drug with respect to receptors for the drug (25, 26). In a landmark *in vivo* study investigating the effect of inhaled drug particle size in patients with asthma using short-acting beta-agonist, the authors observed aerosolized particles of 6- and 3-micron MMAD of monodisperse aerosol achieved a good bronchodilator response as assessed with the forced expiratory volume in one second (FEV_1), whereas the 1.5-micron MMAD aerosols achieved less airways bronchodilation with FEV_1 (10). However, overall the smaller particles achieved greater total lung deposition of drug compared to the larger particles. The authors explained this paradox by noting that the larger particles achieved a better bronchodilator response as the short-acting beta-2 agonist particles were preferentially depositing in the proximal large conducting airways where the beta-2 receptors were associated with a greater density of airway smooth muscle and the endpoint used to asses bronchodilator response, the FEV_1, was relatively more selective for eliciting a response in this lung region compared to the smaller aerosols depositing in the distal smaller conducting airways (10, 27, 28). Indeed, FEV_1 in spirometry is a marker of large airways (29). Since this study, the importance of targeting drug to the small conducting airways has been established, where small-airway dysfunction can be accurately assessed, occurs in obstructive airways diseases of asthma and COPD, and contributes to patient symptom burden and patient outcomes (24, 25). Importantly, inhaler formulations have been engineered to allow commercial devices that can be prescribed to patients that target drug to the large and also small airways, the whole airway tree, and have been shown to improve clinical outcomes compared to large particle therapy (23). In vitro studies have shown that small particles can be exhaled, with values documented as high as 70%; however, these used modes and breathing conditions that did not replicate the human lung and particles that were not therapeutic aerosols. Subsequent in vivo studies using inhaled drug particle show that small therapeutic drug particles are minimally exhaled 4–6% and in similar proportions to large drug particles exhaled 1–3%.

Other physicochemical properties that have been engineered to enhance deposition of inhaled drug particles have been altering the shape of the particles (30), utilizing electrostatic charge on particles (31), using low-density gases, such as helium (32), and changing aerosol properties with low-density large porous particles (33). Particle size may not remain constant as a generated aerosol moves through a delivery system and the respiratory tract. Volatile aerosols may become smaller through evaporation droplets of pure water that evaporate rapidly even under conditions of 100% humidity because of increased pressure inside a small droplet caused by surface tension. For example, a 1-micron droplet of water will evaporate within 0.5 s at room ambient temperature, even under saturated conditions. A 10-micron droplet will evaporate within approximately 1 min (34). It has been shown that the humid airway environment may cause water-soluble hygroscopic drug particles to increase their size causing aerosolized particles to deposit more proximally compared to inert non-hygroscopic particles, yet this phenomenon of "hygroscopic growth" has been shown only using non-pharmacological aerosols in vitro experimentally and in healthy subjects in vivo, but not with therapeutic drug particles in actual patients with respiratory disease (35, 36).

Recent pharmaceutical engineering and developments in drug chemistry have focused on the formulation in pMDIs with respect to their propellants. The Montreal Protocol Treaty in 1989 established the need to eradicate the use of chlorofluorocarbons (CFCs) as propellants in the formulation in pMDIs to protect the ozone layer in the stratosphere, with consequent reformulation of pMDIs with non-ozone depleting propellants, such as hydrofluoroalkanes (HFAs) (37, 38). Reproducible delivery of inhaled drug had to be shown and also clinical outcomes, so some pMDI incorporated improved actuator design, new compatible elastomeric valve components, and changes in the orifice geometry (39, 40). The Kigali amendment of 2019 extends the coverage to HFA and there is innovation in low global warming potential propellants to replace the existing HFA propellants in pMDIs.

Patient Variables

The way each subject breathes also affects drug deposition in the airways. Respiratory frequency, tidal volume, and lung volume will affect the residence time of aerosols in the lungs, and hence the probability of deposition by gravitational and diffusional forces. Changing lung volume will also alter the dimensions of the airways and parenchyma. High level of ventilation during exercise and breath-holding represents extremes of breathing patterns which give rise to markedly different deposition patterns. The results of experiments measuring the effect of breathing pattern on the distribution of aerosol deposition indicate that a) total deposition decreases as breathing frequency increases; b) slow, deep breathing produces uniform deposition throughout the lung, but with little aerosol collection in the large airways; c) rapid, shallow ventilation results in enhanced large-airway deposition and marked heterogeneity in deposition distribution; and d) slow, shallow breathing at high end-expiratory volumes enhanced small-airway deposition (41). In clinics, the most important patient variable affecting inhaled aerosol deposition in the lungs is the breathing maneuver, which influences deposition efficiency and therapeutic efficacy of the inhaled drug particles. For pMDIs and the SMI a slow and steady inhalation over 5 seconds is optimal (42), and patients should be instructed to inhale "slowly, steadily, naturally, deeply and comfortably" [Usmani, personal communication]. It has been shown that a fast, rapid, and quick inhalation decreases aerosol in the lungs and increases oropharyngeal impaction (43). Actuation of pMDIs at the start of the inhalation maneuver during low lung volumes has been shown to enhance the deposition of inhaled drug within the lungs (44). It is important that prior to inhalation from any device that patients lift their chin up, in order to open the airway (45) and also exhale to end tidal functional residual capacity in order to have enough inhaled volume to carry the drug particles in the inspiratory airstream (46). A greater inhaled volume on inspiration allows more aerosolized particles to be effectively deposited within the lungs and carried toward the peripheral airways (47). Instruction to patients to exhale the aerosol via the nose and not the mouth may be beneficial [Usmani, personal communication], where data show the dose of nasal corticosteroid may be significantly reduced in asthma patients with rhinitis (48). In contrast to pMDIs, DPIs are dependent upon the patient's inspiratory flow to operate and require quicker, faster inspiratory inhalation flows to generate sufficient peak inspiratory flow (PIF) and optimally de-aggregate the powdered drug from its carrier molecule and effectively aerosolize the powder into respirable inhaled particles in order to achieve adequate lung deposition (49). The internal resistance of a DPI, and hence the flow required to overcome this resistance, varies with different DPI designs (50). Of note, findings from observational studies (51, 52) suggest that 32–47% of inpatients admitted for exacerbations of COPD demonstrated a suboptimal PIF (<60 L/min) prior to discharge; suboptimal PIF was also reported in 19–78% of stable outpatients with COPD. Taken together, these findings suggest that many patients do not generate sufficient inspiratory force to overcome the resistance of prescribed DPIs. Several independent predictors for suboptimal PIF have been identified, including patient effort, female gender, shorter height, and older age (53, 54).

With the conventional nebulizers the ideal breathing maneuver is relaxed tidal breathing by the patient, and where some new nebulizer devices assess the patient's breathing maneuver and pulse to deliver aerosolized drug only during the inhalation phase leading to a more efficient system and less drug wastage. As discussed, at the end of the inhalation maneuver the breath-hold pause enhances the deposition of inhaled drug in the lungs, with the required airway residence time for the aerosolized particles to make contact with the airway walls through the deposition mechanisms of gravitational sedimentation and diffusion (44).

The configuration of the lungs and airways is important since the efficiency of deposition depends, in part, upon the diameters of the airways, their angles of branching, and the average distances to alveolar walls. Furthermore, along with the inspiratory flow, airway anatomy specifies the local velocity of the airstream, and thus whether the flow is laminar or turbulent. There are inter-intra-species differences in lung morphometry; even within the same individual, the dimensions of the respiratory tract vary with changing lung volume, with aging, and with pathological processes. A highly significant change in the effective anatomy of the respiratory tract occurs when there is a switch between nose and mouth breathing or when the nose is bypassed by a tracheostomy or by an endotracheal tube. The nose has a major role as a collector of inhaled aerosol particles. The combination of a small cross-section for airflow, sharp curves, and interior nasal hairs helps maximize particle impaction. The loss of filtering capacity of the nose may be involved in the exercise-induced asthma. With rising levels of exercise and increasing ventilation, the high-resistance nasal pathway will be abandoned in favor of the low-resistance oral pathway, thus increasing the exposure to more aerosol particles particularly large particles, such as pollen particles. Respiratory diseases markedly influence the distribution of inspired particles. Bronchoconstriction will lead to diversion of flow to non-obstructive airways. With advancing diseases, the remaining healthy airways may be exposed increasingly to inspired particles. Narrowing by inflammation or mucus can increase linear velocities of airflow, enhance inertial deposition, and cause more central deposition patterns. In very sick patients, there may be increases in aerosol deposition which are associated with flow limitation (9, 55). As discussed, the caliber of the patient's airways can affect the lung deposition of inhaled drug, where patients with asthma have less inhaled aerosol deposition in the lungs compared to healthy subjects (9, 55) and following induced bronchoconstriction of the airways (56). However, recently, it has been shown that by altering the pharmaceutical formulation and using drug of smaller particle size may overcome the airway narrowing present in asthma and COPD leading to levels of lung deposition as observed in healthy subjects (57, 58).

Evidence is accumulating that healthcare professionals give inadequate device demonstration to patients as they themselves lack knowledge and instruction in inhaler devices (59). As a consequence, patients are taught incorrectly, or not taught at all, and errors in inhalation technique have been shown to have a direct consequence on worsening disease control and exacerbations in patients, and lead to a greater health economic burden (60). Demonstrating inhaler technique to a patient is an essential part of the management of patients with respiratory disease in outpatients and on the ward as an inpatient and improve disease outcomes (61, 62). Patients should have their inhaler technique checked at every opportunity as it has been shown that correct inhaler technique decreases over time (63). Decreased cognition in elderly patients (64) and relatively poor strength in their hands (65) may lead to an incorrect inhaler technique and focused attention will be needed here with the patient and their caregivers. Simplifying inhaler regimens with the same inhaler device type for concomitant inhaled medications in patients with asthma or COPD can lead to improved clinical outcomes and reduced health care use (66).

FUTURE DIRECTIONS

There is a need for ongoing innovation in inhaled delivery systems to be able to keep up with the rapid advances being seen in in drug discovery, particularly in biopharmaceutics and pharmacogenomics. Inhaled drug delivery systems must be designed in order to achieve better control of aerosolized drug delivered to the airways to be effective in the management of local disease and airway pathology and also for the treatment of systemic disease (67). Indeed, inhaled drug delivery to the lungs is increasingly being investigated as a route for the systemic delivery of therapeutic drug (68). The large surface area of the lungs and vascular supply, particularly the alveolar region, may allow inhaled drug to be effectively absorbed and large molecule peptides and proteins that are unable to be absorbed through the gastrointestinal tract or undergo high metabolic hepatic breakdown may also benefit from the inhalation route in order to achieve a systemic effect. There are clear therapeutic benefits for patients with decreased adverse drug effects and practical advantages of avoidance with needles compared to parenteral therapy.

REFERENCES

1. Lavorini F, Buttini F, Usmani OS. 100 years of drug delivery to the lungs. Handb Exp Pharmacol 2019;260:143–159.
2. Lavorini F, Fontana GA, Usmani OS. New inhaler devices - the good, the bad and the ugly. Respiration 2014;88(1):3–15. DOI:10.1159/000363390
3. Yernault JC. Inhalation therapy: An historical perspective. Eur Respir Rev 1994;4:65–67.

4. Mitchell JP, Berlinski A, Canisius S, et al. Urgent appeal from International Society for Aerosols in Medicine (ISAM) during COVID-19: Clinical decision makers and governmental agencies should consider the inhaled route of administration: A statement from the ISAM Regulatory and Standardization Issues Networking Group. J Aerosol Med Pulm Drug Deliv 2020;33(4):235–238.
5. Darquenne C. Deposition mechanisms. J Aerosol Med Pulm Drug Deliv 2020;33(4):181–185.
6. Verbanck S, Kalsi HS, Biddiscombe MF, et al. Inspiratory and expiratory aerosol deposition in the upper airway. Inhal Toxicol 2011;23(2):104–111.
7. Agnew JE. Physical properties and mechanisms of deposition of aerosols. In: Clarke SW, Pavia D, editors. Aerosols and the lung. London: Butterworths; 1994. p. 49–70.
8. Yu J, Chien YW. Pulmonary drug delivery: Physiologic and mechanistic aspects. Crit Rev Ther Drug Carrier Syst 1997;14:395–453.
9. Melchor R, Biddiscombe MF, Mak VH, et al. Lung deposition patterns of directly labelled salbutamol in normal subjects and in patients with reversible airflow obstruction. Thorax 1993;48:506–511.
10. Usmani OS, Biddiscombe MF, Barnes PJ. Regional lung deposition and bronchodilator response as a function of β2-agonist particle size. Am J Respir Crit Care Med 2005;172:1497–1504.
11. Iwanaga T, Tohda Y, Nakamura S, et al. The Respimat® Soft Mist inhaler: Implications of drug delivery characteristics for patients. Clin Drug Investig 2019;39(11):1021–1030.
12. Johal B, Murphy S, Tuohy J, et al. Plume characteristics of two HFA-driven inhaled corticosteroid/long-acting beta2-agonist combination pressurized metered-dose inhalers. Adv Ther 2015;32(6):567–579.
13. Dreher M, Price D, Gardev A, et al. Patient perceptions of the re-usable Respimatt® Soft Mist™ inhaler in current users and those switching to the device: A real-world, non-interventional COPD study. Chron Respir Dis 2021;18:1479973120986228.
14. Corradi M, Chrystyn H, Cosio BG, et al. NEXThaler, an innovative dry powder inhaler delivering an extrafine fixed combination of beclometasone and formoterol to treat large and small airways in asthma. Expert Opin Drug Deliv 2014;11(9):1497–1506.
15. Vincken W, Levy ML, Scullion J, et al. Spacer devices for inhaled therapy: Why use them, and how? ERJ Open Res 2018;4(2):00065-2018.
16. Lavorini F, Barreto C, van Boven JFM, et al. Spacers and valved holding chambers-the risk of switching to different chambers. J Allergy Clin Immunol Pract 2020;8(5):1569–1573.
17. Verbanck S, Biddiscombe MF, Usmani OS. Inhaled aerosol dose distribution between proximal bronchi and lung periphery. Eur J Pharm Biopharm 2020;152:18–22.
18. Hochrainer D, Hölz H, Kreher C, et al. Comparison of the aerosol velocity and spray duration of Respimat Soft Mist inhaler and pressurized metered dose inhalers. J Aerosol Med 2005;18:273–282.
19. Dhand R. Aerosol plumes: Slow and steady wins the race. J Aerosol Med 2005;18(3):261–263.
20. Sonnenberg AH, Taylor E, Mondoñedo JR, et al. Breath hold facilitates targeted deposition of aerosolized droplets in a 3D printed bifurcating airway tree. Ann Biomed Eng 2021;49(2):812–821.

21. Hillyer EV, Price DB, Chrystyn H, et al. Harmonizing the nomenclature for therapeutic aerosol particle size: A proposal. J Aerosol Med Pulm Drug Deliv 2018;31(2):111–113.
22. Sonnappa S, McQueen B, Postma DS, et al. Extrafine versus fine inhaled corticosteroids in relation to asthma control: A systematic review and meta-analysis of observational real-life studies. J Allergy Clin Immunol Pract 2018;6(3):907–915.e7.
23. Usmani OS. Treating the small airways. Respiration 2012;84(6):441–453.
24. Usmani OS, Dhand R, Lavorini F, et al. Why we should target small airways disease in our management of chronic obstructive pulmonary disease. Mayo Clin Proc 2021;96(9):2448–2463.
25. Usmani OS, Han MK, Kaminsky DA, et al. Seven pillars of small airways disease in asthma and COPD: Supporting opportunities for novel therapies. Chest 2021;160(1):114–134.
26. Usmani OS. Small-airway disease in asthma: Pharmacological considerations. Curr Opin Pulm Med 2015;21(1):55–67.
27. Usmani OS, Biddiscombe MF, Nightingale JA, et al. Effects of bronchodilator particle size in asthmatic patients using monodisperse aerosols. J Appl Physiol 2003;95(5):2106–2112.
28. Biddiscombe MF, Barnes PJ, Usmani OS. Generating monodisperse pharmacological aerosols using a spinning top aerosol generator. J Aerosol Med 2006;19:245–253.
29. Usmani OS. Calling time on spirometry: Unlocking the silent zone in acute rejection after lung transplantation. Am J Respir Crit Care Med 2020;201(12):1468–1470.
30. Hassan MS, Lau RW. Effect of particle shape on dry particle inhalation: Study of flowability, aerosolization, and deposition properties. AAPS PharmSciTech 2009;10(4):1252–1262.
31. Xi J, Si X, Longest W. Electrostatic charge effects on pharmaceutical aerosol deposition in human nasal-laryngeal airways. Pharmaceutics 2014;6(1):26–35.
32. Peterson JB, Prisk GK, Darquenne C. Aerosol deposition in the human lung periphery is increased by reduced-density gas breathing. J Aerosol Med Pulm Drug Deliv 2008;21(2):159–168.
33. Edwards DA, Ben-Jebria A, Langer R. Recent advances in pulmonary drug delivery using large, porous inhaled particles. J Appl Physiol 1998;85:379–385.
34. Mercer TT. Aerosol technology in hazard evaluation. New York (NY): Academic Press; 1973.
35. Finlay WH, Stapleton KW, Chan HK, et al. Regional deposition of inhaled hygroscopic aerosols: In vivo SPECT compared with mathematical modeling. J Appl Physiol 1996;81:374–383.
36. Chan HK, Eberl S, Daviskas E, et al. Changes in lung deposition of aerosols due to hygroscopic growth: A fast SPECT study. J Aerosol Med 2002;15:307–311.
37. Dolovich M. New delivery systems and propellants. Can Respir J 1999;6:290–295.
38. Zeidler M, Corren J. Hydrofluoroalkane formulations of inhaled corticosteroids for the treatment of asthma. Treat Respir Med 2004;3:35–44.
39. Lewis D. Metered-dose inhalers: Actuators old and new. Expert Opin Drug Deliv 2007;4:235–245.

40. Acerbi D, Brambilla G, Kottakis I. Advances in asthma and COPD management: Delivering CFC-free inhaled therapy using Modulite technology. Pulm Pharmacol Ther 2007;20:290–303.
41. Byron PR. Respiratory drug delivery. Boca Raton (FL): CRC Press; 1990. p. 1–38.
42. Laube BL, Janssens HM, de Jongh FH, et al. What the pulmonary specialist should know about the new inhalation therapies. Eur Respir J 2011;37(6):1308–1331.
43. Newman SP, Pavia D, Clarke SW. How should a pressurized beta-adrenergic bronchodilator be inhaled? Eur J Respir Dis 1981;62:3–21.
44. Newman SP, Pavia D, Clarke SW. Improving the bronchial deposition of pressurized aerosols. Chest 1981;80:909–911.
45. Horiguchi T, Kondo R. Determination of the preferred tongue position for optimal inhaler use. J Allergy Clin Immunol Pract 2018;6(3):1039–1041.e3.
46. Ohar JA, Ferguson GT, Mahler DA, et al. Measuring peak inspiratory flow in patients with chronic obstructive pulmonary disease. Int J Chron Obstruct Pulmon Dis 2022;17:79–92.
47. Pavia D, Thomson M, Shannon HS. Aerosol inhalation and depth of deposition in the human lung. The effect of airway obstruction and tidal volume inhaled. Arch Environ Health 1977;32:131–137.
48. Shaikh WA. Exhaling a budesonide inhaler through the nose results in a significant reduction in dose requirement of budesonide nasal spray in patients having asthma with rhinitis. J Investig Allergol Clin Immunol 1999;9(1):45–49.
49. Buttini F, Quarta E, Allegrini C, et al. Understanding the importance of capsules in dry powder inhalers. Pharmaceutics 2021;13(11):1936.
50. Levy ML, Carroll W, Izquierdo Alonso JL, et al. Understanding dry powder inhalers: Key technical and patient preference attributes. Adv Ther 2019;36(10):2547–2557.
51. Ghosh S, Pleasants RA, Ohar JA, et al. Prevalence and factors associated with suboptimal peak inspiratory flow rates in COPD. Int J Chron Obstruct Pulmon Dis 2019;14:585–595.
52. Mahler DA. Peak inspiratory flow rate as a criterion for dry powder inhaler use in chronic obstructive pulmonary disease. Ann Am Thorac Soc 2017;14(7):1103–1107.
53. Duarte AG, Tung L, Zhang W, et al. Spirometry measurement of peak inspiratory flow identifies suboptimal use of dry powder inhalers in ambulatory patients with COPD. Chronic Obstr Pulm Dis 2019;6(3):246–255.
54. Malmberg LP, Rytila P, Happonen P, et al. Inspiratory flows through dry powder inhaler in chronic obstructive pulmonary disease: Age and gender rather than severity matters. Int J Chron Obstruct Pulmon Dis 2010;5:257–262.
55. Kim CS, Kang TC. Comparative measurement of lung deposition of inhaled fine particles in normal subjects and patients with obstructive airway disease. Am Rev Respir Dis 1997;155:899–905.
56. Svartengren M, Anderson M, Philipson K, et al. Individual differences in regional deposition of 6-micron particles in humans with induced bronchoconstriction. Exp Lung Res 1989;15:139–149.
57. De Backer W, Devolder A, Poli G, et al. Lung deposition of BDP/formoterol HFA pMDI in healthy volunteers, asthmatic, and COPD patients. J Aerosol Med Pulm Drug Deliv 2010;23(3):137–148.

58. Virchow JC, Poli G, Herpich C, et al. Lung deposition of the dry powder fixed combination beclometasone dipropionate plus formoterol fumarate using NEXThaler® device in healthy subjects, asthmatic patients, and COPD patients. J Aerosol Med Pulm Drug Deliv 2018;31(5):269–280.
59. Plaza V, Giner J, Rodrigo GJ, et al. Errors in the use of inhalers by health care professionals: A systematic review. J Allergy Clin Immunol Pract 2018;6(3):987–995.
60. Usmani OS, Lavorini F, Marshall J, et al. Critical inhaler errors in asthma and COPD: A systematic review of impact on health outcomes. Respir Res 2018;19(1):10.
61. van Beerendonk I, Mesters I, Mudde AN, et al. Assessment of the inhalation technique in outpatients with asthma or chronic obstructive pulmonary disease using a metered-dose inhaler or dry powder device. J Asthma 1998;35:273–279.
62. Capstick TG, Azeez NF, Deakin G, et al. Ward based inhaler technique service reduces exacerbations of asthma and COPD. Respir Med 2021;187:106583.
63. Klijn SL, Hiligsmann M, Evers SMAA, et al. Effectiveness and success factors of educational inhaler technique interventions in asthma & COPD patients: A systematic review. NPJ Prim Care Respir Med 2017;27(1):24.
64. Allen SC. Competence thresholds for the use of inhalers in people with dementia. Age Ageing 1997;26:83–86.
65. Armitage JM, Williams SJ. Inhaler technique in the elderly. Age Ageing 1988;17:275–278.
66. Usmani OS, Hickey AJ, Guranlioglu D, et al. The impact of inhaler device regimen in patients with asthma or COPD. J Allergy Clin Immunol Pract 2021;9(8):3033–3040.e1.
67. Biddiscombe MF, Usmani OS. Is there room for further innovation in inhaled therapy for airways disease? Breathe (Sheff) 2018;14(3):216–224.
68. Gonda I. Systemic delivery of drugs to humans via inhalation. J Aerosol Med 2006;19:47–53.

2 Goals of Pharmacotherapy for Asthma and COPD

Donald A. Mahler and Marc Miravitlles

CONTENTS

INTRODUCTION

The goals of inhaled therapy for patients with asthma and chronic obstructive pulmonary disease (COPD) have evolved from enhancing lung function to improving clinical outcomes. This paradigm shift was largely a result of two factors: 1) an emphasis on patient experiences and symptoms related to their airway disease and exacerbations and 2) the development of instruments and scales to quantify symptoms, especially dyspnea, quality of life, exercise capacity, and exacerbations. Currently, patient advocacy organizations, investigators, thought leaders, professional organizations, and pharmaceutical companies prioritize these patient-reported outcomes (PROs).

Evidence from phases II, III, and IV clinical trials has demonstrated that various inhaled therapies improve PROs in those with asthma and COPD. Such information has enabled expert panels and global leaders to provide specific pharmacologic recommendations targeted to achieve the goals of therapy for these airway diseases. Ideally, the stated goals from national and international experts/organizations assist health care professionals (HCPs) in addressing three decisions required when prescribing inhaled therapy (Figure 2.1): 1) Do I select a short-acting and/or one or more long-acting bronchodilators? 2) What class(es) of medication is/are appropriate or best for the individual patient–beta-agonist, muscarinic antagonist, and/or corticosteroids? 3) Which delivery system is appropriate or best for the individual patient?

The following information reviews the stated goals of pharmacotherapy by major organizations and/or countries for individuals with asthma and COPD. Although the overall goals of pharmacotherapy apply regardless of the delivery system (inhaled, injected, intravenous, or swallowed), the inhaled approach is preferred for individuals with asthma and COPD.

ASTHMA

The Global Initiative for Asthma (GINA) is the most widely recognized professional source for prescribing therapies for individuals with asthma (1). In addition, Expert Panel Reports of the United States National Asthma Education and Prevention Program provide guidelines for the diagnosis and management of children and adults with asthma (2). Asthma experts sponsored by the Japanese Society of Allergology published guidelines for adults with

DOI: 10.1201/9781003269014-2

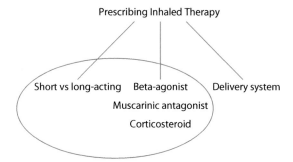

Figure 2.1 When prescribing inhaled therapy, health care professionals (HCPs) must make three decisions—two involve selecting the medication(s) (circled), while the other relates to selecting the delivery system.

asthma living in Japan (3). Furthermore, the Department of Veterans Affairs partnered with the Department of the Defense in the United States to develop a clinical practice guideline for the primary care management of asthma (4). Information on recommended goals for the treatment of asthma found in these four documents is presented below in alphabetical order and is summarized in Table 2.1.

Department of Veterans Affairs/Department of Defense

In 2019, a panel of multidisciplinary experts published a clinical practice guideline based on a systematic review of clinical and epidemiological evidence related to asthma (4). The guideline is intended for the "primary care management of asthma" with the main goal being "Asthma Control." Specific criteria are listed for assessing whether a patient's asthma is "Controlled" or "Not Controlled" based on two components: Impairment and Risk (Table 2.1). Impairment is assessed by daytime symptoms, night time awakening, interference with normal activities, short-acting beta-agonist (SABA) use, and the Asthma Control Test. Risk is assessed by the number of exacerbations requiring oral systemic corticosteroids and treatment-related adverse effects.

Expert Panel Report 3 of the National Asthma Education and Prevention Program

In 1989, the National Asthma Education and Prevention Program was created to address asthma issues in the United States. Three Expert Panel Reports have been published – in 1991, 2002, and 2007. According to the Expert Panel Report 3, the goal of therapy is "Control of asthma," based on two components: Reduce impairment and Reduce risk. Specific items for these components are listed in Table 2.1. In 2020, a focused update on six priority topics was published based on systematic reviews using the Population, Intervention, Comparator, and Outcomes (PICO) format (2).

GINA

GINA was established following a workshop in 1993 organized by the National Heart, Lung, and Blood Institute and the World Health Organization. GINA

Table 2.1: **Goals of Pharmacotherapy in Asthma**

Source (Alphabetical Order)	Goals
Department of Veterans Affairs and Department of Defense (4)	Asthma control
	Impairment
	<ul><li>Daytime symptoms</li><li>Nighttime awakening</li><li>Interference with normal activities</li><li>SABA use for symptom control</li><li>Asthma control test score</li></ul>
	Risk
	<ul><li>Exacerbation requiring oral steroids</li><li>treatment-related adverse effects</li></ul>
Expert Panel Report 3 of the National Asthma Education and Prevention Program (2)	Control of asthma
	Reduce Impairment
	<ul><li>Prevent symptoms</li><li>Infrequent use of inhaled SABA</li><li>Maintain (near) normal pulmonary function</li><li>Maintain normal activity levels</li><li>Meet patient/family expectations of asthma</li></ul>
	Reduce risk
	<ul><li>Prevent recurrent exacerbations</li><li>Prevent loss of lung function</li><li>Provide optimal pharmacotherapy</li></ul>
Global Initiative for Asthma (1)	Asthma control
	Symptom control
	<ul><li>Daytime asthma symptoms</li><li>Night waking due to asthma</li><li>SABA reliever for symptoms more than twice/week</li><li>Any activity limitation due to asthma</li></ul>
	Risk factors for poor asthma outcomes
	<ul><li>Various factors listed in document</li></ul>
Japanese Guidelines for Adult Asthma (3)	Asthma control
	<ul><li>Asthma symptoms (in daytime or at night)</li><li>Use of reliever</li><li>Limitations of activities, including exercise</li><li>Lung function</li><li>Diurnal (weekly) variation in PEF</li><li>Exacerbation</li></ul>

Abbreviations: PEF = peak expiratory flow; SABA = short-acting beta-agonist.

has published a "Global Strategy for Asthma Management and Prevention," that has been updated annually since 2002 (1). The GINA Science Committee currently consists of 16 experts from 11 different countries. The committee used a 2009 definition of asthma control, "The extent to which the features of asthma are apparent or have reduced or eliminated by controller treatment" (5). Asthma control is considered over the past four weeks based on two domains: symptom control and risk of adverse outcomes, particularly exacerbations (1). The document proposed that the level of asthma symptom control be classified as, "Well controlled," "Partly controlled," and "Uncontrolled," based on specific items for asthma listed in Table 2.1.

Japanese Guidelines for Adult Asthma

In 2020, 12 asthma experts representing the Japanese Society of Allergology updated a Japanese guideline for adult asthma published three years earlier (3). The new guideline noted that the prevalence of asthma in Japan had increased from 1% to 10% or higher in children and to 6% to 10% in adults since the 1960s. The stated aims of asthma treatment are "Symptom control" and "Avoidance of future risks." Based on six specific items for asthma control listed in Table 2.1, asthma can be assessed as "Well controlled," "Insufficiently controlled," and "Poorly controlled."

COPD

The Global Initiative for Obstructive Lung Disease (GOLD) is the most recognized source for prescribing inhaled therapies for individuals with COPD (6). The GOLD program was initiated in 1998 with the first report being issued in 2001. Subsequent revisions have been made based on levels of evidence with yearly updates since the fourth major revision in 2017. In addition, the American Thoracic Society and Canadian Thoracic Society have each published clinical practice guidelines on pharmacotherapy for patients with COPD (7, 8). Experts on COPD in Spain have updated published guidelines on pharmacologic management (9). Information on recommended goals for the treatment of COPD in these four documents is presented in alphabetical order below and is summarized in Table 2.2.

American Thoracic Society

In 2020, the American Thoracic Society (7) published a clinical practice guideline to address specific clinically important questions regarding pharmacologic management of COPD. The introduction stated that the aims of pharmacologic treatment of COPD are to 1) improve quality of life; 2) control symptoms; and 3) reduce the frequency of exacerbations. Six clinical questions were posed using the PICO format. The expert panel used the Grading of Recommendations Assessment, Development, and Evaluation (GRADE) approach for each clinical question. Two questions examined therapy for "patients with COPD who complained of dyspnea or exercise intolerance," whereas a third question addressed "patients who experience advanced refractory dyspnea."

Canadian Thoracic Society

In 2019, a panel of six respirologists, three clinicians/epidemiologists, two primary care physicians, and one pharmacist in Canada updated a clinical practice guideline from a position statement that was published in 2017 (8).

Table 2.2: **Goals of Pharmacotherapy in COPD**

Source (Alphabetical Order)	Goals
American Thoracic Society (7)	Improve quality of life Control symptoms Reduce the frequency of exacerbations
Canadian Thoracic Society (8)	Improve shortness of breath Improve exercise tolerance Improve physical activity Prevent exacerbations
Global Initiative for Chronic Obstructive Lung Disease (6)	*Reduce symptoms* • Relieve symptoms • Improve exercise • Improve health status *Reduce risk of exacerbations* • Prevent disease progression • Prevent and treat exacerbations • Reduce mortality
Spanish COPD Guideline (9)	Alleviate symptoms Reduce frequency/severity of exacerbations Improve quality of life Extend survival

The authors proposed that their guideline was "a step toward personalized therapy based on increasing individual characterization." The approach to pharmacotherapy aligns treatment decisions with "symptom burden" and the "risk of future exacerbations" as shown in Table 2.3.

The recommended goals of therapy are detailed in two PICO questions. PICO 1 addressed optimal use of inhaled and oral pharmacologic maintenance therapies for "symptom burden." with the expressed intent to "improve shortness of breath, exercise tolerance, physical activity, and health statues." PICO 2 addressed "preventing acute exacerbations in stable COPD patients."

GOLD

The GOLD Scientific Committee consists of 18 experts from nine countries. The document provides two major goals for treatment of stable COPD: 1) reduce

Table 2.3: **Approach to Pharmacotherapy Proposed by the Canadian Thoracic Society (8)**

	Mild	Moderate and Severe	
Symptom burden			
Dyspnea (mMRC scale)	1	≥ 2	
CAT	< 10	≥ 10	
Risk of Exacerbation		*Low*	*High*
(# in past year)		Low: ≤ 1 not requiring ED visit or hospitalization High = > 2 treated with antibiotic and/or corticosteroid or >1 requiring ED visit or hospitalization	

Abbreviations: CAT = COPD assessment test; ED = Emergency Department; mMRC = modified Medical Research Council scale.

symptoms and 2) reduce risk. There are three specific outcomes for each goal as shown in Table 2.2 (6). Initial pharmacological treatment is recommended based on categorizing each patient into one of four quadrants (A, B, C, and D) according to low or high symptoms as measured on the modified Medical Research Council scale or the COPD Assessment Test (CAT) and low or high risk of exacerbations according to the number and type of events in the past year.

After initial therapy is prescribed, a management cycle of [Review → Assess → Adjust → Review] is recommended to evaluate whether treatment goals have been obtained. If not, then the HCP should consider the predominant treatment trait—dyspnea or exacerbations—to decide on any changes in pharmacologic treatment.

Spanish COPD Guideline

In 2021, the Spanish COPD guideline (GesEPOC) for the pharmacological treatment of stable patients with COPD were updated (9). First published in 2012, the current GesEPOC is the fourth update. The document stated that it was the first clinical guideline on COPD to propose treatment based on clinical phenotypes (9). According to the authors, the guideline offers a more individualized approach to COPD treatment tailored according to the clinical characteristics of patients and their level of complexity. The 2021 guideline assesses five new PICO questions using GRADE methodology (9).

Once a diagnosis of COPD is made, patients are stratified as being either *low or high risk* based on three criteria as described in Table 2.4. Initial pharmacological treatment is guided by symptoms in low-risk patients and by clinical phenotype in high-risk individuals. The document states that there is greater need for therapy in the higher risk level.

This guideline introduces the concept of control of COPD as an objective of treatment for the first time (10). Control of COPD consists of two components: clinical impact (how much the disease interferes with the daily life of patients) and clinical stability (the lack of impairment over time and the absence of exacerbations) (10). The variables used to measure impact and stability are shown in Table 2.4. A patient is considered to be controlled when the disease has a low impact and stable.

Table 2.4: Risk Stratification and Control Criteria Proposed in the 2021 Spanish COPD Guideline (9)

Clinical Evaluation	With Adjustment for $FEV_1\%$	
Low clinical impact (At least three of the four criteria should be fulfilled)		
	$FEV_1 \geq 50\%$	$FEV_1 \leq 49\%$
• Dyspnea	0–1	0–2
• Rescue medication	≤3 times/week	
• Sputum color	White or absent	
• Physical activity	≥30 min/day	
Clinical stability (Both criteria should be fulfilled)		
• Subjective perception	Same or better	
• Exacerbations in the last three months	None	
Control	Low impact + Stability	

Abbreviation: FEV_1 = forced expiratory volume in one second.

DISCUSSION

"Asthma Control" is the primary goal of pharmacotherapy for individuals with asthma as described in four recently published documents (Table 2.1). *Impairment/symptoms* and the *risk of future exacerbations* are the two major components that reflect whether a person's asthma is controlled or not. Both the Department of Veterans Affairs/Department of Defense (4) and the Expert Panel Report 3 (2) use *impairment* to include symptoms, ability to perform normal activities, and use of an inhaled short-acting beta-agonist (SABA) bronchodilator and the heading *risk* to include exacerbations. GINA (4) lists *symptom control* to capture the same items as those included with *impairment*. The Japanese Guidelines (3) enumerate symptoms, use of reliever inhaler, and exacerbations as three of six items that reflect "Asthma Control."

Symptom relief and *reducing the risk of future exacerbations* are the major goals of pharmacotherapy for individuals with COPD as described in the four recently published documents (Table 2.2). Improvement in quality of life is included in the American Thoracic Society document (7) as well as in the Spanish Guideline (9) as a specific objective, whereas improved health status is listed under the heading "Reduce Symptoms" in the GOLD Strategy (6). Improvements in exercise tolerance and physical activity are additional goals proposed by the Canadian Thoracic Society (8), while "Improve exercise" is included under the heading "Reduce symptoms" in the GOLD strategy (6). Both the GOLD strategy (6) and the Spanish Guideline (9) propose that "Reduce mortality/extend survival" are further aims of therapy for patients with COPD.

Although the overall goals of pharmacotherapy are remarkably similar for patients with asthma and COPD, the conceptual approach is generally different. Whereas "disease control" is the dominant theme of pharmacotherapy for asthma, only the Spanish COPD guideline recommends this concept for individuals with COPD (9). In 2014, Soler-Cataluña *et al.* (10) first proposed "clinical control in COPD" defined as "The long-term persistence of a situation of low clinical impact." Subsequently, prospective studies demonstrated that lack of control of COPD, as defined in the Spanish guideline (9), is very sensitive to clinical changes in patients (11) and is a very good predictor of poor outcomes, including exacerbations, hospital admissions, or mortality (12). Furthermore, the concept of "disease control" in COPD is supported by the findings of an online survey in which 445 individuals with COPD indicated that "symptom control" was the top information priority when searching the internet about their condition (13).

Despite the general difference in approach noted above, specific objectives of pharmacotherapy are consistent for both asthma and COPD—relief of symptoms and reducing the risk of a future exacerbation (Tables 2.1 and 2.2). Certainly, dyspnea, or breathing difficulty, is the most common symptom experienced by patients with airway obstruction. Coughing is another frequent complaint in both asthma and COPD and may be the presenting symptom in either condition. Exacerbations are a major burden for patients with asthma and COPD that contribute to morbidity and, at times, mortality and add substantially to health care costs. Thus, reducing the risk of a future exacerbation is a shared goal for both asthma and COPD.

Numerous inhaled medications have been shown to be beneficial by improving symptoms and by reducing the risk of an exacerbation in patients with asthma and COPD (1, 6). To be effective, the medication must be inhaled deep into the lower respiratory tract to act on airway receptors. Selecting one or more medications in an appropriate inhaled delivery system and then instructing patients with asthma and COPD on correct inhaler technique are critical to achieve the goals of pharmacotherapy (14).

REFERENCES

1. Reddel HK, Bacharier LB, Bateman ED, et al. Global initiative for asthma strategy 2021: Executive summary and rationale for key changes. Am J Respir Crit Care Med 2022;205:17–35.
2. Expert Panel Working Group of the National Heart, Lung, and Blood Institute (NHLBI) administered and coordinated National Asthma Education and Prevention Program Coordinating Committee. 2020 focused updates to the asthma management guidelines: A Report from the National Asthma Education and Prevention Program Coordinating Committee Expert Panel Working Group. J Allergy Clin Immunol 2020;146:1217–1270.
3. Nakamura Y, Tamaoki J, Nagase H, et al. Japanese guidelines for adult asthma 2020. Allergol Int 2020;69:519–548.
4. VA/DoD clinical practice guideline for the primary care management of asthma. https://www.healthquality.va.gov/guidelines/cd/asthma. Accessed 21 Sept 2022.
5. Reddel HK, Taylor DR, Bateman ED, et al. An official American Thoracic Society/European Thoracic Society statement: Asthma control and exacerbations: Standardizing endpoints for clinical asthma trials and clinical practice. Am J Respir Crit Care Med 2009; 180:59–99.
6. Global initiative for Chronic Obstructive Lung Disease. Global strategy for the diagnosis, management, and prevention of chronic obstructive pulmonary disease. 2022 report. https://goldcopd.org/2022-gold-reports-2. Accessed 21 Sept 2022.
7. Nici L, Mammen MJ, Charbek E, et al. Pharmacologic management of chronic obstgructive pulmonary disease. An official American Thoracic Society clinical practice guideline. Am J Respir Crit Care Med 2020;201;e56–e69.
8. Bourbeau J, Bhutani MN, Hernandez P, et al. Canadian Thoracic Society clinical practice guideline on pharmacotherapy in patients with COPD – 2019 update of evidence. Can J Respir Crit Care Sleep Med 2019;3:210–232.
9. Miravitlles M, Calle M, Molina J, et al. Spanish COPD guidelines (GesEPOC) 2021: Updated pharmacological treatment of stable COPD. Arch Bronchoneumol 2021;58:69–81.
10. Soler-Cataluña JJ, Alcazar-Navarrete B, Miravitlles M, et al. The concept of control of COPD in clinical practice. Int J Chronic Obstr Pulm Dis 2014;9:1397–1405.
11. Soler-Cataluña JJ, Alcazar B, Marzo M, et al. Evaluation of changes in control status in COPD: An opportunity for early intervention. Chest 2020;157:1138–1146.
12. Miravitlles M, Sliwinski P, Rhee CK, et al. Changes in control status of COPD over time and their consequences: A prospective international study. Arch Bronconeumol 2021;57(2):122–129.
13. Mahler DA, Cerasoli F, Della L, et al. Internet health behaviors of patients with chronic obstructive pulmonary disease and assessment of two disease websites. Chronic Obstr Pulm Dis 2018;5:158–166.
14. Usmani OS, Hickey AJ, Guranlioglu D, et al. The impact of inhaler device regimen in patients with asthma or COPD. J Allergy Clin Immunol Pract 2021;9:3033–3040.

3 Pressurized Metered-Dose Inhalers (pMDI)

Donna D. Gardner and Sandra G. Adams

CONTENTS

INTRODUCTION

One of the most important aspects of living with an obstructive lung disease such as asthma or chronic obstructive pulmonary disease (COPD) is empowering patients to manage their disease every day with correct and consistent use of the prescribed inhaled medications. The most common device used to administer aerosolized medication day-to-day for acute symptom relief and for maintenance treatment is the pressurized metered-dose inhaler (pMDI). Similar to all inhalers, the pMDI requires proper inhaler technique in order to ensure effective medication delivery deep into the lungs. The pMDI requires patients to inhale slowly and to appropriately coordinate their breathing with inhaler actuation to ensure effective medication delivery (1). Incorrect use of the pMDI is a significant barrier to appropriately treating and managing asthma and/or COPD. Correct use of the pMDI is essential.

WHAT IS A pMDI AND WHAT DOES IT LOOK LIKE?

A pMDI is a multi-dose device that generates an aerosol to deliver medication to the airways. The concept is about 65 years old, with a Meshberg metering valve device that was originally designed for dispensing perfume using a glass container. Since the introduction of this original device to the market, the pMDI has evolved to

DOI: 10.1201/9781003269014-3

COMPONENTS

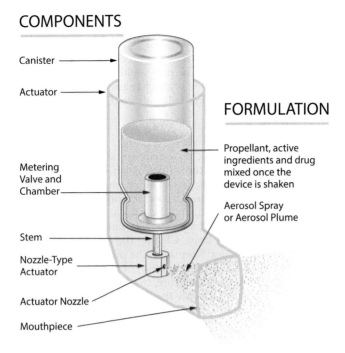

Figure 3.1 Illustrated are components of the metered-dose inhaler depicting a suspension of the propellant, active ingredients, and drug after being shaken (pink with blue dots), as well as the components of the canister and actuator as labeled.

provide effective delivery of inhaled medication to the lungs (Figure 3.1). The active medication(s) and the propellant are sealed in the pMDI aluminum canister which rests within a plastic actuator. A closed pressurized reservoir within the canister protects the ingredients from degradation, contamination, moisture, and light. When the device is shaken appropriately, the medication is suspended or dissolved in the propellant. Pressing/actuating the canister allows a known, predefined volume of propellant and micronized drug to be released from the metering valve and chamber (2, 3). The propellant drives the drug through the actuator nozzle and into the air. The propellant droplets evaporate immediately, resulting in an aerosol spray or an aerosol plume, which is ready for inhalation through the mouthpiece (4).

The current pMDIs contain hydrofluoroalkane (HFA) propellants. The HFAs deliver an aerosol plume with a low-impact force, yet have a smaller delivery orifice, resulting in a slowly delivered aerosol plume. These factors facilitate inhalation deep into the lungs and produce less mouth and throat irritation when the pMDIs are used correctly. The HFA carries the drug in solution. The dose may feel and taste different than the "old" pMDIs, which used chlorofluorocarbons (CFCs) and were discontinued by an international agreement under the Montreal Protocol. The HFA pMDI aerosol contains a wide range of particle sizes (0.5–10 μm) (5). Despite these small particle sizes, less than 30% of the dose reaches the lower respiratory tract even if the inhalation technique is flawless (6, 7). This is because a significant portion (more than 70%) of the medication deposits in the

21

back of the throat (oropharynx) (6, 7). A slower inhalation reduces deposition of the drug in the oropharynx and deep breathing facilitates deeper deposition in the lungs where the medication is most useful (5).

All pMDIs in the United States are now required to have a dose counter, like the ones pictured in Figure 3.2. The pMDI with dose counter indicates the number of puffs left in the device and often changes color when nearing the last few doses. When the last puff is taken/administered, it is important to throw the device away.

BREATH-ACTUATED INHALER (BAI)

The breath-actuated inhaler (BAI), beclomethasone dipropionate (QVAR) Redihaler™, is the only breath-actuated pMDI available in the United States. Other medications are available as BAI in other countries. These BAI devices overcome the need for the hand-breath coordination. The dose is ready for inhalation when the cap is opened, and the patient breathes in through the mouthpiece. The patient's inspiratory flow generated by inhalation triggers the release of a unit-dose of the drug. Closing the cap prepares the device for the next dose. The Redihaler™ replaced the previous beclomethasone (QVAR) formulation. With the BAI technology, a very low inspiratory flow is required to trigger the device; therefore, the BAI should not be shaken or primed. If the patient were to shake the device, there is a chance the device will actuate the dose into the air because of the sensitivity of the trigger mechanism. In addition, this device should not be used with a valved holding chamber or spacer. This breath-actuated inhaler technology improves particle stability, provides a consistent dose, and has more efficient lung deposition. Finally, this device may be useful for patients who have difficulty using a traditional pMDI due to reduced strength in the hands, debilitating diseases, or cognitive issues that make hand-breath actuation and coordination challenging (1).

WHAT MEDICATIONS ARE AVAILABLE IN pMDIs?

Currently, there are various short-acting and long-acting individual and/ or combinations of the three different classes or types of medications: short-acting beta-agonist (SABA), short-acting muscarinic antagonists (SAMA, or anticholinergic agents), inhaled corticosteroids (ICSs), and combination medications that include a long-acting beta-agonist (LABA) and ICS, LABA and long-acting muscarinic antagonist (LAMA), ICS, LABA, and LAMA (see Figure 3.2), and ICS and SABA (not pictured).

HOW TO USE THE pMDI

Educating patients using the actual device (from the patient or in placebo form) and the "teach back" or "return demonstration" technique is essential to ensure that patients have the appropriate knowledge and skills to successfully manage their obstructive lung disease. Effective education empowers patients to manage their disease and increases their awareness of the danger signs indicating clinical deterioration or exacerbation (8). The healthcare professional (HCP) must regularly assess and reassess medication adherence and inhaler technique at each patient encounter in order to optimize disease management and control (8, 9). Furthermore, with advances in digital monitoring technology and communication, the use of telemedicine and education can be woven into the care of patients using the pMDI (see Chapter 7). Digital monitoring systems with text messages or reminder systems can improve adherence to medication use.

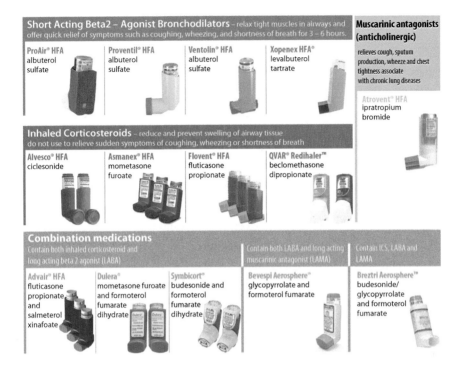

Short Acting Beta2 – Agonist Bronchodilators – relax tight muscles in airways and offer quick relief of symptoms such as coughing, wheezing, and shortness of breath for 3 – 6 hours.

ProAir® HFA albuterol sulfate	Proventil® HFA albuterol sulfate	Ventolin® HFA albuterol sulfate	Xopenex HFA® levalbuterol tartrate

Muscarinic antagonists (anticholinergic)

relieves cough, sputum production, wheeze and chest tightness associate with chronic lung diseases

Atrovent® HFA ipratropium bromide

Inhaled Corticosteroids – reduce and prevent swelling of airway tissue do not use to relieve sudden symptoms of coughing, wheezing or shortness of breath

Alvesco® HFA ciclesonide	Asmanex® HFA mometasone furoate	Flovent® HFA fluticasone propionate	QVAR® Redihaler™ beclomethasone dipropionate

Combination medications

Contain both inhaled corticosteroid and long acting beta 2 agonist (LABA)			Contain both LABA and long acting muscarinic antagonist (LAMA)	Contain ICS, LABA and LAMA
Advair® HFA fluticasone propionate and salmeterol xinafoate	Dulera® mometasone furoate and formoterol fumarate dihydrate	Symbicort® budesonide and formoterol fumarate dihydrate	Bevespi Aerosphere® glycopyrrolate and formoterol fumarate	Breztri Aerosphere™ budesonide/ glycopyrrolate and formoterol fumarate

Figure 3.2 All inhaled medications and classes which are available for use in the metered-dose inhaler throughout the United States are depicted.

CLOSED-LIP TECHNIQUE

The pMDIs can be inhaled using the "closed lip" technique or with a valved holding chamber (sometimes referred to as a "spacer"). When using the "closed lip" technique, firing (or actuating) the device too early or too late may completely undermine delivery. Early firing, even by 0.5 seconds, before the onset of inspiration can reduce deposition of aerosol in the lung by 34% (10). However, waiting until after the first half of inspiration to fire the device typically reduces lung deposition by 41% (10).

The pMDI should be inhaled slowly and steadily following a maximal expiration. The inhaler should be actuated just *after* the onset of inspiration if using the "closed lip" technique. The total inhalation should take about 3–5 seconds. Finally, the breath should be held for about 6–10 seconds after full inhalation.

CLOSED-LIP TECHNIQUE: STEPS TO PROPERLY USE THE pMDI

1. Take the cap or dustcover off the inhaler mouthpiece and look inside the mouthpiece to make sure nothing is inside the mouthpiece (like a gum wrapper or coin that might be accidentally inhaled into the airways).

2. Shake the inhaler for approximately 5 seconds (see manufacturer's instructions for each device because this may not be necessary for some HFA pMDIs).

3. Before the first use and if not used for a period of time, *prime* the pMDI by holding the mouthpiece away from you and pushing the top of the canister down, releasing one puff of medication into the air. Repeat these steps if needed, according to the manufacturer's instructions.

TO USE THE pMDI

1. Sit or stand up straight.

2. Check the dose counter to make sure there are doses available.

3. Remove the cap or dustcover off the inhaler mouthpiece and look inside the mouthpiece to make sure nothing is inside the mouthpiece (like a gum wrapper or coin) that might be accidentally inhaled into the airways.

4. Hold the pMDI upright with the mouthpiece at the bottom and the canister on top.

5. Shake the device for at least 5 seconds *before* each use.

6. Face away from the device, breathe out to empty your lungs.

7. Place the pMDI mouthpiece between your lips and teeth.

8. Seal your lips tightly around the mouthpiece.

9. Start breathing slowly in and immediately push down on the top of the inhaler *once*, to release the medication or aerosol spray.

10. Continue breathing in very slowly for 3–5 seconds or until your lungs are full of air.

11. Remove the inhaler from your lips and hold your breath for up to 10 seconds or as long as possible.

12. Breathe out slowly, away from the device.

13. Wait for 20–60 seconds if another puff of medicine is needed and then repeat the steps above, starting with step 8. Shake the device for 5 seconds before each use.

14. When finished using the pMDI, always replace the cap or dustcover.

To reduce the risk of thrush if the pMDI contains an inhaled corticosteroid, rinse your mouth and gargle with water and SPIT the water OUT—Do NOT swallow this water—to reduce the risk of thrush.

See the video for reference: https://youtu.be/2_dLTUtKlWE

Note: The pMDI plastic holder should be cleaned with a damp cloth or with "swishing" in water to prevent occlusion of the canister nozzle. Do NOT place the canister in water.

OPEN-MOUTH TECHNIQUE

The open-mouth technique for MDI inhalation is no longer recommended by many experts (11). The amount of force and velocity with which the medication came out of the older CFC formulations was high, resulting in significant deposition of the medication in the mouth. Therefore, with the old CFC formulations, actuating the MDI while holding it approximately two finger breadths away from the lips made sense and helped reduce the unwanted oropharyngeal deposition. Now, the HFA formulations have completely replaced the CFC formulations. Therefore, the open-mouth technique is no longer felt to be useful or needed since the HFA formulation comes out of the MDI with less force and velocity, resulting in more medicine reaching the lungs and less being deposited in the oropharynx.

VALVED HOLDING CHAMBERS (VHCs) AND SPACER DEVICES WITH pMDIs

Valved holding chambers (VHCs) and spacer devices have been developed in order to eliminate problems with coordination. The chambers reduce the velocity of the aerosol being delivered and generally increase the medication delivery to the peripheral airways. Because the VHC has a one-way valve, it is not necessary to begin the breath prior to actuating the pMDI, thereby removing the need for hand-breath coordination. Similar to the closed-lip technique, a slow inspiration through the VHC after actuation of the pMDI is required to deliver the medicine deep into the lungs. Finally, a breath-hold lasting 6–10 seconds is still expected when using the pMDI with VHC.

THE VALVED HOLDING CHAMBER AND SPACER DEVICES WITH pMDI: STEPS FOR PROPER USE

1. Take the cap or dustcover off the inhaler mouthpiece and look inside the mouthpiece to make sure nothing is inside (like a gum wrapper or coin) that might be accidentally inhaled into the airways.

2. Shake the inhaler for approximately 5 seconds (see manufacturer's instructions for each device).

3. Before the first use and if not used for a period of time, *prime* the pMDI by holding the mouthpiece away from you and push the top of the canister down, releasing one puff of medication into the air. Repeat these steps if needed, according to the manufacturer's instructions.

TO USE THE pMDI WITH VHC

1. Sit or stand up straight.

2. Check the dose counter on the canister to make sure there is a dose available.

3. Take the cap or dustcover off the inhaler mouthpiece and the VHC mouthpiece. Look inside the mouthpieces to make sure nothing is inside the mouthpiece (like a gum wrapper or coin) that might be accidentally inhaled into the airways.

4. Hold the pMDI upright with the mouthpiece at the bottom and the canister on top.

5. Shake the inhaler for approximately 5 seconds (see manufacturer's instructions for each device).

6. Place the mouthpiece of the pMDI into the rubber-sealed end of the VHC.

7. Turn away from the pMDI and VHC and breathe out to empty your lungs.

8. Place the VHC mouthpiece between your lips and teeth.

9. Seal your lips tightly around the VHC mouthpiece.

10. Press down on the top of the pMDI *once* to actuate the medication and release the aerosol spray.

11. Start breathing in slowly over 3–5 seconds until your lungs are full of air.

12. Remove the VHC mouthpiece from your lips.

13. Hold your breath for up to 10 seconds or as long as possible.

14. Breathe out slowly, away from the device.

15. Wait for 20–60 seconds if another puff of medicine is needed and then repeat the steps above, beginning with Step 8. Shake the inhaler for approximately 5 seconds.

16. When finished with using the pMDI, always replace the cap or dustcover.

To reduce the risk of thrush if the pMDI contains an inhaled corticosteroid, rinse your mouth, gargle with water, and SPIT the water OUT—Do NOT swallow this water.

See the VIDEO for reference: https://youtu.be/03EeVhhUajc

TO USE A BREATH-ACTUATED INHALER (BAI)

1. Make sure the cap or dustcover is closed over the mouthpiece.

2. Look at the dose counter to see there is a dose available.

3. Sit or stand up straight.

4. Hold the inhaler upright.

5. Remove the cap or dustcover from the BAI mouthpiece until you hear a "click" sound. This indicates the dose is loaded and ready for you to inhale.

6. Turn away from the mouthpiece of the inhaler and breathe out to empty your lungs.

7. Place the mouthpiece between your lips and make a tight seal (make sure fingers do not cover the "airvents" on top of the canister).

8. Breathe in deeply through the mouth. As you inhale, the BAI will release a puff of medicine.

9. Remove the device from your mouth.

10. Hold your breath for up to 10 seconds or as long as you are able.

11. Slowly exhale.

12. Close the cap or dust cover firmly over the mouthpiece and make sure it "clicks" to close the cap tightly.

13. If a second dose is needed, wait for 20–60 seconds, then repeat the steps, beginning with Step 4. Hold the inhaler upright.

See the VIDEO for reference: https://youtu.be/wxF2aXfW_DE

Note: The BAI should never be primed, shaken, or used with a VHC or spacer. This device may be an alternative for patients with arthritis if they are not able to actuate the traditional pMDI. The BAI is approved for children aged 4 years and older.

WHEN TO USE A pMDI

The pMDI may be used for rescue/as a quick relief medication or as a maintenance/controller medication or both, depending on the medication in the device. Medications classified as short-acting beta 2 agonist (SABA) bronchodilators and the short-acting muscarinic antagonists (SAMA) (Figure 3.2) are used as a quick relief medication when the patient is experiencing signs and symptoms associated with obstructive lung diseases, such as wheezing, cough, shortness of breath, and/or chest tightness. The medications classified as inhaled corticosteroids (ICSs) are used as maintenance/controller medications and have been recently recommended to be used as a quick relief medication (to replace the SABA) when combined with either formoterol or albuterol for patients with asthma (8, 12). After using any medication with an inhaled corticosteroid, it is important to remind the patient to rinse and gargle with water and spit to reduce the risk of oral thrush. *Candida* is a fungus that often causes thrush. This fungus is a normal type of flora that lives in our mouths. When the ICS particles are deposited in the mouth and on the tongue, the immune system within the oropharynx weakens and allows the fungus to grow and spread throughout the mouth, which is called oral thrush. The lesions of thrush are often sore and usually appear as small white patches on the inner cheeks, tongue, roof of mouth, and throat. Some patients report having a "cotton-like" dryness in their mouth and some lose their sense of taste. Others with thrush experience pain while eating or swallowing and may have cracking or redness at the corners of the mouth. Therefore, to markedly reduce the risk of thrush, it is imperative to rinse and gargle with water and spit out the water to remove the deposited medication from the mouth and throat. However, if a patient develops thrush, treatment with antifungal lozenges, liquid, or pills is usually very effective.

ADVANTAGES OF THE pMDI
The Patient
Advantages of using a pMDI include the following: it is portable, lightweight, compact, and requires short treatment time. The pMDI does not require a high inspiratory flow, the medication dose is the same with each actuation, and many combinations of medications are available within one device. Furthermore, the advantages of using a pMDI with a VHC include significantly improved patient coordination, higher lung deposition of medication, and reduced deposition of medication in the oropharynx and mouth. In addition, the required inspiratory effort to inhale the medication is lower when a VHC is used. Similar to the pMDI, the BAI's advantages include being portable, lightweight, compact, and requiring short treatment time. The BAI also has multiple doses and a combination of medications in one device. One major advantage of the BAI over the pMDI is that the BAI does not require the coordination of inhalation and actuation.

The Healthcare Professional
The advantages of the pMDI from the point of view of the HCP include those mentioned in the patient advantages above. In addition, various combinations of medications are available in the pMDI formulation, allowing for improved likelihood that the preferred classes of medications will be available on insurance plans and hospital formularies.

DISADVANTAGES AND COMMON ERRORS WHEN USING THE pMDI
The Patient
The disadvantages of the pMDI include the hand-breath coordination needed when using this device in order to successfully inhale the medication deep into the lungs and that the medication may deposit in the back of the mouth/throat instead of being delivered to the airways deep within the lungs.

Also, to actuate the device, the patient must push down on the canister, which may be difficult for some with significant hand arthritis. Some common errors when using pMDI occur in many patients with hand/finger pain, who may turn the device upside down to actuate with their thumb. However, the device will not work when upside down because the propellants are gravity dependent and only work when the device is upright.

There is frequently confusion in the use of pMDI due to the plethora of devices on the market and the similar appearance of devices, such as the Respiclick and Digihaler, which are dry powder inhalers but appear like the pMDI and BAI devices. Patients may not properly understand how to use the pMDI, including how to prepare and handle the device before each dose. Other common mistakes including breathing in too quickly, which is associated with depositing more medicine in the oropharynx rather than deep in the lungs. In addition, if the medication is used without a VHC, critical errors often result in ineffective delivery of medication into the lungs. These major errors include the following: Actuating the canister too early (before starting the inhalation), stopping/ceasing inspiration upon release of the medication aerosol, and actuating the device too late in the inhalation cycle. In addition, if the breath-hold does not occur, the drug may be expelled and not delivered to the airways. Any error in any step may lead to inadequate drug delivery to the lung (13). Several studies have shown that patients with COPD and asthma commonly misuse the pMDI in real life (10, 14–16).

Furthermore, the disadvantages of using the pMDI with VHC or spacer are that it is not as portable as the pMDI alone, the VHC requires regular cleaning, and there are additional costs associated with purchasing the VHC. Lastly, the BAI has some disadvantages as well, which include accidental release of the medication into the air if the patient inadvertently shakes the device with the cap open and that there may be some confusion with the BAI because people are not familiar with this device.

The Healthcare Professionals

There is confusion in the use of the pMDI among HCP due to the plethora of devices on the market, and the HCP may not properly understand all the steps required to properly use the inhaler. Mastering pMDI use involves preparing and handling the device as well as ensuring optimal inhaler technique. A single error in any step of the inhaler technique may lead to suboptimal drug delivery to the lung (13). Even when patients are given detailed instructions and are appropriately able to demonstrate the technique back to the educator (called return demonstration), the intricacies and the number of steps required may result in one or more critical inhaler technique errors. In addition, frequently, any given patient's inhaler technique deteriorates over time, and requires reassessing inhaler technique at every encounter and reviewing the proper steps, whether in person or via a telehealth visit.

CONCLUSIONS

Successful management of the symptoms and complications of obstructive lung diseases requires teamwork between the healthcare professionals and the patients in order to improve health outcomes. Adherence and proper use of inhaled medications for obstructive lung diseases via traditional pMDI and breath-actuated pMDI require careful and repeated instruction, assessment, and reassessment at every patient-HCP encounter. HCPs need to exhibit vigilance to detect errors in inhaler technique, whether subtle or obvious, that may reduce drug delivery and overall effectiveness of the inhaled medications in patients with obstructive lung diseases.

REFERENCES

1. Usmani O. Choosing the right inhaler for your asthma or COPD patient. Ther Clin Risk Manag 2019;15:461–472.
2. Salvi S, Shevade M, Aggarwal A, et al. A practical guide on the use of inhaler devices for asthma and COPD. J Assoc Physicians India 2014;15:326–338.
3. Tena A, Clara P. Deposition of inhaled particles in the lungs. Arch Bronchoneumol 2012;48(7):240–246.
4. Chierici V, Cavalieri L, Piraino A, et al. Consequences of not-shaking and shake-fire delays on the emitted dose of some commercial solution and suspension pressurized metered dose inhalers. Expert Opin Drug Deliv 2020;17(107):1025–1039.
5. Sanchis J, Corrigan C, Levy M, et al. Inhaler devices from theory to practice. Respir Med 2013;107:495–502.
6. Newman S, Weisz A, Clarke S. Improvement of drug delivery with a breath actuated pressurised aerosol for patients with poor inhaler technique. Thorax 1991;46(10):712–726.
7. Leach C, Colice G. A pilot study to assess lung deposition of HFA-beclomethasone and CFC-beclomethasone from a pressurized metered dose inhaler with and without add-on spacers and using varying breathhold times. J Aerosol Med Pulm Drug Deliv 2010;23(6):355–361.
8. Reddel HK, Bacharier LB, Bateman ED, et al. Global initiative for asthma strategy 2021 - Executive summary and rationale for key changes. Am J Respir Crit Care Med 2022;205(1):17–35.
9. Global Initiative for Chronic Obstructive Lung Disease. Global strategy for the diagnosis, management, and prevention of chronic obstructive pulmonary disease. 2023 report. [cited 2022 Dec 21]. Available from: https://goldcopd.org/2023-gold-report-2
10. Kaplan A, Price D. Matching inhaler devices with patients: The role of the primary care physician. Can Respir J 2018;2018:9473051.
11. Labiris NR, Dolovich MB. Pulmonary drug delivery. Part II: The role of inhalant delivery devices and drug formulations in therapeutic effectiveness of aerosolized medications. Br J Clin Pharmacol 2003;56(6):600–612.
12. Papi A, Chipps BE, Beasley R, et al. Albuterol-budesonide fixed-dose combination rescue inhaler for asthma. N Engl J Med 2022;386:2071–2083.
13. Usmani O, Lavorini F, Marshall J, et al. Critical inhaler errors in asthma and COPD: A systematic review of impact on health outcomes. Respir Res 2018;19(10):1–20.
14. Lavorini F, Usmani O. Correct inhalation technique is critical in achieving good asthma control. Prim Care Respir J 2013;22(4):385–386.
15. Sanchis J, Gich I, Pedersen S, et al. Systematic review of errors in inhaler use. Has patient technique improved over time? Chest 2016;105(2):394–406.
16. Molimard M, Raherison C, Lignot S, et al. Chronic obstructive pulmonary disease exacerbation and inhaler device handling: Real-life assessment of 2935 patients. Eur Respir J 2017;49:1601794.

4 Spacers and Valved Holding Chambers

Rajiv Dhand and Myrna B. Dolovich

CONTENTS

INTRODUCTION

Pressurized metered-dose inhalers (pMDIs) became commercially available in 1956 and patients with asthma and chronic obstructive pulmonary disease (COPD) rapidly adopted them as the preferred modality for personalized treatment (1) and they remain immensely popular to this day (2). The unique attributes of convenience of use, perceived ease of use of pMDIs, and portability are major factors for their widespread use among patients. However, soon after the introduction of pMDIs two significant problems became apparent, namely, the inability of many patients to synchronize their inhalation with actuation of the pMDI and the high velocity of the emitted aerosol spray that resulted in high oropharyngeal deposition of drug (3, 4). Several devices were developed to overcome these twin problems, including complex breath-activated devices which initiated drug delivery only when the patient developed adequate negative inspiratory pressure to simple tubes (5, 6) and chambers (7, 8) that added space between the patient's mouth and the pMDI.

The introduction of spacers and valved holding chambers (VHCs) in the 1980s as accessory devices for pMDI delivery of aerosolized drugs proved to be of major benefit for many adult and pediatric patients. Coordinating actuation of the pMDI to release the dose of medication with inhalation of the fast-moving aerosol cloud emitted was challenging for the majority of adult and all pediatric users of pMDI treatments for asthma (9); the attachment of a spacer or VHC to the pMDI allowed patients to manage these two maneuvers, thereby obtaining their aerosolized medication more easily. The design, properties, and function of a number of spacers and VHCs will be discussed in this chapter, describing the differences between products and the many factors and outcome measures that should be considered when choosing a spacer/VHC for patients.

Spacer devices, also known as "add-on devices," "extension devices'" "accessory devices," or "valved holding chambers," are available in a variety of dimensions and design features (Figure 4.1). The drug emitted by a pMDI forms an aerosol cloud

DOI: 10.1201/9781003269014-4

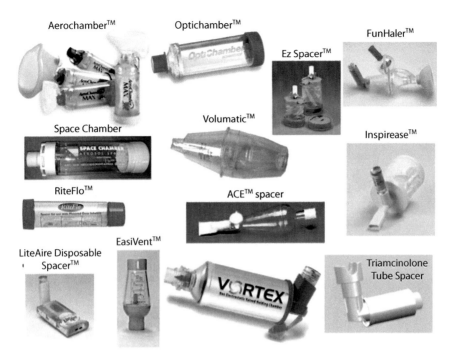

Aerochamber™   Optichamber™

FunHaler™

Ez Spacer™

Volumatic™

Space Chamber

Inspirease™

RiteFlo™   ACE™ spacer

EasiVent™

LiteAire Disposable
     Spacer™

Triamcinolone
Tube Spacer

Figure 4.1 Photograph showing a variety of commercially available spacers and VHCs for attachment with pMDIs. Spacers and VHCs have several designs and are available in a variety of sizes (see text for details).

within the spacer. A VHC has a one-way valve to hold the aerosol in the chamber after pMDI actuation for a finite time and permits airflow into, but not out of, the patient's mouth (Figure 4.2). In the "reverse-flow" design, the pMDI placed close to the mouth is actuated in a direction away from the patient into a spacer from which the patient inhales, thereby doubling the length that the aerosol travels (10). Spacers reduce oral deposition while VHCs can reduce both oral deposition and the need for precise synchronization between actuation and inhalation (Table 4.1).

HOW SPACERS/VHCs WORK

Spacers and VHCs have several effects on the aerosol produced by pMDIs (Figure 4.2). First, the high velocity of the drug aerosol emitted from the pMDI actuator is reduced due to the impaction and loss of large particles to the chamber walls, along with losses resulting from the increased distance/time between actuation and inhalation by the patient. Second, the deposition of drug in the oropharynx is reduced because larger particles, which have the greatest inertia at high velocity and which are most likely to deposit in the mouth or throat, impact, or sediment due to gravity within the spacer. The residual aerosol or "respirable" portion of the original aerosolized drug, contained in smaller particles <5μm in diameter, remains available for inhalation and deposition in the lung. Finally, the use of a VHC holds the remaining aerosol within the chamber for a finite time after pMDI actuation, reducing the need for precise coordination between actuation of the pMDI and inhalation of the remaining aerosol. Some VHCs incorporate an audible feedback signal to warn against too rapid an inspiratory flow; in other devices this signal is used as a guide to promote the optimal inhalation flow rate

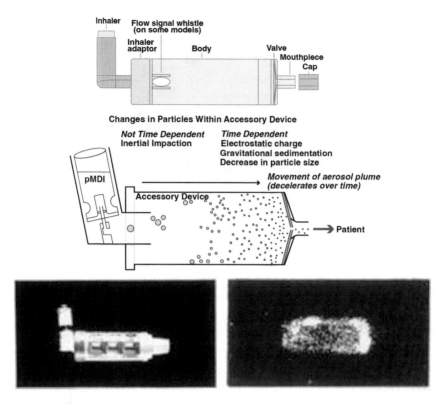

Figure 4.2 Illustration showing the components of a VHC connected to a pMDI (top panel). In the AeroChamber, the reed that signals flow is incorporated into the outer ring of the rubber backpiece. The changes in the aerosol plume produced by the pMDI as it traverses the chamber of the VHC are shown (middle panel). The aerosol plume released from the pMDI travels at varying velocities, dependent on the formulation (propellants, excipients, and drug) (11). At high velocities, the plume impacts on the valve and may fold back on itself, traveling to the back of the VHC. This movement likely results in particle deposition on the VHCs inner surface, reducing the available aerosol for inhalation as well as altering the particle size of the available aerosol (12). As inhalation begins, the aerosol plume again reverses direction, moving toward the mouth with a decreased forward velocity. During this finite time, partial evaporation of the propellant(s) continues, increasing the fine particle fraction of the available aerosol and further decreasing the overall particle size of the aerosol. Two images (lower panel) show the AeroChamber™ VHC, with a pMDI inserted into the rubber backpiece on the left and on the right, a gamma camera scan post one actuation from a radioactive bronchodilator aerosol. The high concentration of "hot spots" on the inspiratory valve (white area) represents particles from the pMDI that would otherwise impact in the oropharynx and larynx. (Modified from M Dolovich. Physical principles underlying aerosol therapy. Journal of Aerosol Medicine 1989; 2(2): 171–186. Reproduced with permission.)

Table 4.1: Spacers/VHCs: Function and Effect

Effect of Spacer/VHC	Clinical Impact
Reduces need for coordination between inhalation and actuation	Beneficial for 20–50% of patients using pMDIs who have difficulty with coordinating inhalation with actuation (13)
Selective removal of larger particles by impaction on spacer walls	Reduction in size of the aerosol particles exiting the spacer/VHC leading to more uniform deposition of aerosol in the healthy lung (14, 15)
Decreased spray velocity and reduced oropharyngeal deposition	Reduced local and systemic side-effects (e.g., tremor, oral thrush) (4, 16)
Feedback signal to guide optimal inhalation flow	Increase in lung deposition as a proportion of nominal dose (8, 17–19)

Abbreviations: pMDI = pressurized metered-dose inhaler; VHC = valved holding chamber.

with pMDI use. The use of spacers also reduces the bad taste associated with oral deposition of some drugs (triamcinolone acetonide, flunisolide) and propellants and mitigates the "cold-Freon effect" in some patients (20).

AEROSOL DELIVERY TO THE LUNG

Reduction in the forward velocity of the aerosol as it traverses the spacer/ VHC coupled with the decrease in particle size of the aerosol reduces drug deposition in the oropharynx by several folds (4, 17). Dolovich and co-workers (21) reported the clinical evaluation of a VHC that was the early version of the AeroChamber, a 145-mL cylinder which incorporated a rubberized opening into which the pMDIs mouthpiece actuator (or "boot") could fit regardless of pMDI actuator shape. Using a [99m]technetium radiolabeled pMDI aerosol they showed a reduction in throat deposition, from 65% with the pMDI alone to 6.5% with the AeroChamber in bronchitic subjects (21). Notably, *peripheral* lung deposition of aerosol improved and there was more uniform lung deposition with use of the VHC in the healthy subjects, but not in those with chronic bronchitis, underscoring the influence of airways obstruction on aerosol deposition in the lung. Moreover, in the COPD subjects, lung deposition was almost identical for the pMDI alone (17.4%) versus the pMDI with holding chamber (18.0%) when the values were corrected for tissue adsorption of radioactivity (21).

Newman and co-workers, employing radiolabeled aerosol and a 750-mL spacer device with a one-way inhalation valve (Nebuhaler, Astra Pharmaceuticals), corroborated the dramatic reduction in aerosol losses in the throat from ~80% with the pMDI alone, but they noted a corresponding increase in aerosol loss in the chamber (~56%) (8). In that study (8), there was a significant increase in the fraction of the total dose to the lungs with a valved large volume spacer (20.9%) compared to a pMDI alone (8.7%). Besides the device characteristics, other factors, such as the age-specific breathing pattern and airway morphology, also influence lung deposition of aerosol from spacer devices (19).

FACTORS INFLUENCING DRUG DELIVERY FROM SPACERS AND VHCs

The design of spacers and VHCs employ 3 basic concepts—the open tube (OT) design, the reservoir or holding chamber (HC) design, and the reverse-flow (RF) design, in which the pMDI, placed close to the mouth—is fired in the direction away from the patient (10, 22, 23).

Some spacers integrate flow restrictors to control the patient's inspiratory flow and incorporate mechanisms to coordinate inhalation with pMDI actuation (e.g., Optihaler, Healthscan Products, Cedar Grove, NJ). Other spacers/VHCs provide

Table 4.2: **Factors Influencing Performance of Spacers and VHCs**

pMDI related	Spacer/VHC related	Patient related
Volume of aerosol cloud	Dimensions (size, shape)	Age
Concentration of aerosol	Presence of valves (inspiratory, expiratory)	Tidal volume
Aerosol velocity	Materials (plastic, metal, non-conducting polymers)	Inspiratory flow
Metering valve dimension	Flow indicators	Coordination with actuation; dose of API inhaled
Excipients in formulation	pMDI actuator design	Breath-hold
Formulation (e.g., type of propellant, vapor pressure)	Vents for air entrainment	Presence of airway obstruction
	Durability of device	Use of facemask or mouthpiece

Abbreviations: API = active pharmaceutical ingredient; pMDI = pressurized metered-dose inhaler; VHC = valved holding chamber.

an audible warning when the patient inhales too fast (e.g., Aerosol Cloud Enhancer, DHD Diemolding Healthcare Division, Canastota, NJ; AeroChamber, Monaghan Medical Corporation, Plattsburgh, NY; Inspirease, Schering Corporation, Kenilworth, NJ). Collapsible plastic bags are used to increase the volume of some spacers but can degrade if alcohol is an excipient in the formulation. However, several issues associated with pMDIs are not resolved simply by adding a spacer/VHC because a pMDI and spacer/VHC combination creates a unique device whose performance is influenced by a variety of factors (Table 4.2).

Several different spacer/VHCs, based on the three concepts mentioned above and with volumes ranging from 15 to 750 ml, are currently available (Table 4.3). Figure 4.1 illustrates some devices that are currently commercially available.

Table 4.3: **Volume of Some Commonly Employed Spacers/VHCs**

Type of spacer/VHC	Trade Name	Volume (ml)
Open Tube Spacers	Microspacer	15
	Azmacort	113
	Ellipse	230
Holding Chambers	OptiChamber	140
	AeroChamber	145
	Vortex	180[a]
	Rondo	270
	Babyhaler	350
	Nebuhaler	700
	Volumatic	750
Reverse-Flow Design	Optihaler	70
	Ace	170
	Inspirease	700

Abbreviations: VHC = valved holding chamber.

[a] Approximate volume based on the dimensions of the chamber.

The impaction of particles is related to their mass, velocity, and distance traveled on release from the pMDI. Therefore, particles emerging from the pMDI actuator at a higher velocity have an increased tendency to impact on the inner surface of the spacer. This factor is especially important for small volume spacers, as drug losses on the walls of such spacers lead to a significant reduction in total drug output from the spacer (24, 25).

Early studies demonstrated that more aerosolized drug would likely be available for deposition in the lung when using longer and wider tubes attached to pMDIs (5). However, the portability of a larger, wider spacer becomes an issue for ambulatory patients. In a VHC, the amount of "respirable" aerosol was shown to increase with some formulations (7, 26). Usually, a spacer/VHC increases the fine particle fractions (FPFs) of the aerosol released into the device and this may translate into a greater fine particle mass of drug available for inhalation (27, 28), if the emitted dose is higher with a larger VHC design. However, a higher efficiency of drug delivery, especially with inhaled corticosteroids, needs to be balanced with the potential to cause greater side effects (29–32), and this outcome may not be looked upon favorably by regulatory agencies.

The portability and ease of use of an accessory device could influence patients' compliance with treatment. Except for the Inspirease, spacers/VHCs employed in ambulatory patients are non-collapsible; thus, pMDI and accessory spacers/VHCs are larger and heavier than the pMDI alone. Corr and colleagues found that spacers with a chamber volume of 145 ml width 9 cm, and length of 11 cm had a high efficiency for delivering aerosol from a pMDI (7). Likewise, drug output from accessory devices with a volume between 145 and 250 mL was found to be comparable to that from the pMDI alone (25). Accessory devices with volumes of ~ 700 ml improve pulmonary deposition of aerosol (8), but their large size makes them cumbersome for patients to carry. Although devices with smaller chamber volumes (≤120 mL) are more portable, they have the potential to significantly reduce drug delivery (25). Thus, accessory devices with intermediate volumes (~150 mL) appear to provide the best combination of performance and portability.

Patients should be instructed to release one actuation of the pMDI into the spacer or holding chamber per inhalation as inhalation after actuation of multiple doses into the spacer markedly reduces total drug available due to increased wall loses (33–35). In a large volume spacer/VHC, particles are evenly distributed throughout inhalation because the aerosol cloud becomes static before inhalation. In contrast, the aerosol cloud remains turbulent in small-volume spacers, and they may deliver an initial burst of concentrated aerosol followed by comparatively aerosol-free air (36) that could drive the aerosol further down the bronchial tree. In a large volume spacer, a single actuation of the pMDI may not deliver all the drug particles during one inhalation compared with a smaller volume spacer (37).

The low-resistance, one-way valve situated behind the mouthpiece (Figure 4.2) in VHCs retains the aerosol for a finite time within the device until the patient inhales and allows VHCs to be used with tidal breathing as well as with a single, deep inspiration. The inhalation valve must withstand the initial pressure from pMDI actuation yet have a sufficiently low resistance to open readily on inhalation, especially when using a VHC for infants and children (38–40). In VHCs, drug losses due to sedimentation occur during the interval between actuation and inhalation, while losses due to impaction are flow dependent and occur non-uniformly, mostly in the distal part of the spacer/VHC (41), and on the inhalation valve upon pMDI actuation.

Some VHCs also incorporate an exhalation valve. The exhalation valve should be a low resistance valve to allow comfortable exhalation, but with sufficient resistance to prevent re-entry of the aerosol into the VHC. A large dead space between inspiratory and expiratory valves could reduce mean dose delivery (42, 43). The last part of each inhalation is trapped between the inspiratory and expiratory valve and may be lost with exhalation. This dead space in the delivery system constitutes an increasing fraction of the tidal volume in infants and children below the age of 4 years and tends to produce an inverse relationship between age and the dose of drug delivered (43, 44).

Valves may become jammed if soiled or damaged and require cleaning or replacement of the device if that doesn't resolve the issue. The valve material may degrade over a year of use due to the propellants in the pMDI formulation, losing its ability to respond to inspiratory and expiratory pressures.

ELECTROSTATIC CHARGE

Aerosols emitted from pMDIs have an intrinsic electrostatic charge (45) which varies with different formulations (46–48). VHCs made from non-conducting polymers also acquire surface electrostatic charge during manufacture, packaging, and storage (49). Deposition of aerosol particles on the walls of electrostatic spacers due to electrostatic attraction reduces the drug dose and half-life of the aerosol in the spacer (33, 50).

O'Callaghan and colleagues (33) and Barry and O'Callaghan (50) first reported that drug output was more than two-fold higher when the spacer was coated with a thin film of an antistatic spray before actuation of the pMDI compared to the non-coated device. The antistatic lining also negated the reduction in drug output which occurred when there was a 20-sec delay between actuation of the pMDI and a simulated patient breath. Similarly, improvement in albuterol output delivered by a volumatic spacer in which the static charge was decreased was reported by Dewsbury and colleagues (51). Priming the spacer with multiple doses from a pMDI can also increase drug deposition in the lungs (52), but it could reduce the number of doses available for therapy. Electrostatic charge is reduced by build-up of a thin layer of drug and surfactant that are components of the aerosol spray. This coating is washed off by rinsing the spacer and drug output diminishes until the protective coating builds up again (33–35). Priming is not recommended for those HFA pMDIs that do not contain surfactant; priming the spacer may have a variable effect on drug output and is wasteful of medication (53).

Electrostatic charge on the inner walls of plastic spacers can significantly influence drug output (33, 50). Washing a plastic spacer, newly removed from its packaging and drip drying, can decrease the electrostatic charge in the unused spacer. But drying must occur before the initial use, which is not always convenient for patients. Drying the spacer by wiping it with a cloth will increase the electrostatic charge and is not recommended. The electrostatic charge, and the drug output, will vary over time because of priming of the spacer with use and additional variations introduced by periodically washing the spacer that is needed for hygienic reasons and to prevent build-up of powder on the inspiratory valve from altering the properties of the valve. Thus, washing and subsequent priming of the spacer could result in repeated variations in the amount of drug output from the spacer (54).

The effects of electrostatic charge can be overcome by either lightly coating the internal surface of the VHC or spacer with an antistatic spray, or spraying it with an antistatic lining, washing with a dilute solution (1:5,000) of household detergent and air drying for 24 hours, or by using a metallic spacer (55, 56). The material used to coat the spacer should be non-toxic if inhaled by the patient and approved by the Food and Drug Administration for human use. If a non-static spacer is used, the potential for higher dose delivery may require dose modifications of some drugs, such as inhaled corticosteroids, that produce significant local or systemic side effects (29–32).

Use of a non-static spacer could have several benefits:

- Increased drug output, this effect could be particularly beneficial for expensive medications (demonstrated with several drugs and spacers). After detergent washing, drug output from intermediate volume (145 ml) spacers/VHCs was shown to be equivalent to large volume spacers (750 ml) in both in-vitro and in-vivo studies (29, 55–58). Similarly, after application of an anti-static coating, differences in drug output between large volume and intermediate volume spacers were less evident with HFA-pMDIs compared to the CFC formulations (15, 59, 60). These observations could be explained by the reduced velocity of the aerosol plume emitted by the HFA-pMDIs compared to CFC-pMDIs, thus resulting in fewer wall losses (61).

- Protection of aerosol dose when there is a delay between actuation and inhalation (as in infants and children).

- Greater uniformity in drug output over time (not shown conclusively).

- Enhanced therapeutic effects (62). The response to albuterol administered with a pMDI during periods of nocturnal bronchospasm was reported to increase mean percentage predicted FEV_1 values more with an antistatic spacer than with a non-conducting spacer (63). Likewise, in a real-world retrospective study a cohort using an antistatic spacer reported a decrease in the annualized rate of moderate to severe exacerbations, prolonged time to first moderate to severe exacerbation and reduced incidence of visits to the Emergency Department and hospitalizations compared to those using any non-antistatic spacer over a period of 1 year (64).

However, the use of non-static spacers could also be associated with certain adverse effects:

- Higher drug output has the potential for greater local/systemic side effects (29–32)

- The coefficient of variation in the drug output from the spacer may not decrease, i.e., the drug output per dose showed significant variation even in coated spacers (42, 43).

SWITCHING pMDIs AND SPACERS ALTERS DRUG DELIVERY

The addition of spacers and VHCs to pMDIs contributes to variability in delivery of drug in both children and adults (14, 25, 28, 65–69). The combination of a pMDI with an accessory device has unique characteristics because different pMDIs have different vapor pressures, aerosol velocities, and aerosol volumes (70). Various spacers/VHCs are not interchangeable with different pMDIs because different spacers/VHCs have variable effects on total drug output, fine particle dose, and dose protection against incoordination and actuation (25, 71–73). Significant variations in drug output occur when the drug canister is removed from its native actuator and then coupled with a third-party actuator built into the spacer (74). The dimensions of the valve stem in the universal actuator are usually larger than that of the native mouthpiece actuator of the pMDI. This issue is mainly a problem for spacers integrated into ventilator circuits but is also relevant for portable, reverse-flow spacers and VHCs. Beyond the variability in aerosol characteristics introduced by using a spacer/VHC, it is worth considering that clinical outcomes associated with use of these devices are influenced by other factors, including patient preference, technique of use, and adherence to treatment (75). A systematic review highlighted the high frequency of incorrect inhaler use reported over a span of 40 years. Surprisingly, incorrect use of pMDIs persisted with addition of inhalation chambers and adults committed errors with pMDIs and chambers more frequently than children (76). In view of these findings, real-world studies are needed to evaluate the clinical use and benefit and the cost-effectiveness of using spacers/VHCs with pMDIs in patients with asthma and COPD.

USE OF SPACERS/VHCs IN CHILDREN

There are two main problems related to spacer use in children (77). Because of the low tidal volume, it takes several breaths for a child to clear the aerosol from the chamber and during this time, aerosol passively disappears from the reservoir by sedimentation due to gravity. Second, the inspiratory valve used in holding chambers must operate at low inspiratory flow rates observed in children and ensure unidirectional air flow from the holding chamber with exhalation outside the device. Otherwise, the aerosol retained in the holding chamber may be blown away during exhalation.

A single slow and deep breath followed by a breath-hold is ideal (22, 78). If the patient is unable to take a deep breath, tidal breathing through the device may be similarly effective in children (79). Other investigators have suggested that tidal breathing may not be as effective as a deep inspiration (18). If tidal breathing is employed, the pMDI should be activated at the beginning of a tidal inhalation (80). In very young children with low tidal volumes, fewer breaths are needed to clear the aerosol from a smaller volume compared to a large volume spacer/VHC. Physicians should consider the spacer volume/tidal volume ratio when selecting an appropriate device for their young patients. Too high a spacer volume/tidal volume ratio limits the amount of drug a child might inhale from the spacer and reduces efficacy of the therapy. Three-to-five tidal breaths are usually recommended before significant losses of useful aerosol are incurred.

VHCs can be used to administer pMDI medications to neonates and very young children with appropriately fitting facemasks (81, 82). Snug but comfortable fit of the mask to the cheeks is important to avoid leakage of aerosol-laden air around the facemask edges (81) and minimization of facemask dead space (83) is critical to avoid re-breathing through the mask, thereby not drawing aerosol from the VHC (77).

RECOMMENDATIONS FOR USE

The use of spacers/VHCs is recommended by several national and international guidelines, especially for children using inhaled corticosteroids with pMDIs (84, 85). However, these guidelines are less frequently implemented in clinical practice. For example, surveys show that less than 50% of patients with asthma and COPD have spacers/VHCs and many patients presenting to an emergency room with exacerbations of asthma or COPD have not used these devices (86–88). Use of spacers/VHCs may be more common among patients who have a primary care physician or those who have been hospitalized for an acute exacerbation of asthma or COPD (88). Moreover, a significant proportion of patients exhibit errors in the use of pMDIs and spacers (89). Infants, children below the age of 3 years, the elderly and frail individuals who are unable to coordinate inhalation with actuation of the pMDI, those with compromised comprehension or manual dexterity, and those experiencing acute attacks of asthma or COPD could benefit from use of spacers/VHCs with their pMDIs (90–95). In young children (ages 2 months to 5 years) a low-cost home-made modified 500-mL plastic bottle spacer was shown to be as effective as a commercially available spacer for treatment of acute airway obstruction as measured by improvements in clinical score and pulmonary function (96). Most elderly patients can use pMDIs and spacers

Table 4.4: **Technique for Using a Spacer/VHC**

1. Sit or stand up straight with the chin up and neck slightly extended
2. Shake the pMDI and remove its cap
3. If using a VHC check that the valve(s) is moving appropriately
4. Fit the pMDI into the spacer/VHC with the canister up and hold it in an upright position
5. Keep the pMDI-spacer/VHC assembly in a horizontal position on one hand holding the pMDI with the other hand supporting the mouthpiece end of the spacer/VHC
6. Breathe out as far as comfortable
7. Place the mouthpiece of the spacer/VHC between the teeth and seal the lips around it. If a facemask is used, place it gently but firmly over the nose and lips to make a tight seal
8. Start a slow breath in and immediately press the inhaler once. Continue to breathe in slowly for 3–4 seconds until the lungs are full
9. Hold the breath for 10 seconds or for as long as is comfortable
10. While holding the breath take the spacer/VHC out of the mouth (or lower the mask)
11. Exhale into room air. Do not exhale into the spacer/VHC
12. Repeat the sequence of steps 2–11 for additional doses
13. Take the pMDI out of the spacer/VHC, and replace the cap on the pMDI and the mouthpiece of the spacer/VHC
14. Rinse the mouth and gargle after inhalation of a corticosteroid

Abbreviations: pMDI = pressurized metered-dose inhaler; VHC = valved holding chamber.

effectively (97). The addition of a large facemask can facilitate aerosol delivery in the elderly patient, particularly if keeping the spacer/VHC mouthpiece in the mouth proves difficult. However, adult patients of all ages who exhibit appropriate technique of pMDI use may not derive greater bronchodilation from the use of a pMDI and spacer/VHC compared to a pMDI alone (98, 99).

Use of spacers/VHCs in ambulatory patients adds to the cost of treatment compared with pMDIs alone and the increased permutations of the delivery device could be confusing for some patients. Significant variability in drug output occurs with pMDI and different spacers/VHCs and some pMDI and spacer/VHC combinations may reduce drug delivery (23, 24, 36, 58, 72, 99, 100).

COMPARISON OF EFFICACY OF pMDIs AND SPACERS/VHCs WITH DRY POWDER INHALERS (DPIs) AND NEBULIZERS

pMDIs and VHCs are convenient for administering bronchodilators to infants and children, and to adults during acute exacerbations of asthma or COPD. Several systematic reviews and meta-analyses have concluded that administration of bronchodilators with a pMDI and VHC combination is equally effective as a nebulizer or a DPI in both children and adults with acute asthma (101). A lower incidence of side effects with the pMDI and VHC in patients with acute asthma receiving bronchodilator therapy may be an added advantage (102–106).

INHALATION TECHNIQUE FOR SPACERS/VHCs

The recommended technique for using a spacer/VHC is summarized in Table 4.4.

- Multiple doses must never be actuated into the spacer/VHC. Each actuation should be followed by inhalation of the aerosol (33).

- Multiple actuations into the spacer/VHC before inhalation create turbulence and significantly reduce the respirable fraction of the aerosol (24, 33, 35, 50).

- There should be minimal delay between actuation of the pMDI and breathing in through the spacer/VHC. Too long a delay (≥ 10 sec) significantly reduces the dose available for inhalation (24, 25, 33, 50, 107, 108).

- Coordination between inhaling and actuation of the pMDI is required even while using a spacer/VHC. Actuation of the pMDI without inhaling or during exhalation may further reduce drug delivery (25).

- A single slow and deep inhalation followed by a breath-hold is optimal (22, 78).

- Spacers/VHCs are not generic devices and should not be used interchangeably with other pMDIs (70).

MAINTENANCE OF SPACERS/VHCs

Manufacturers of spacers/VHCs provide guidance for maintenance. Clearly, poor maintenance of spacers/VHCs could influence the efficiency of aerosol delivery (71).

Spacers/VHCs must be washed before their first use and cleaned periodically because they can be contaminated with microorganisms. Bacterial contamination of spacers appears to be fairly common. Contamination with *Pseudomonas aeruginosa, Staphylococcus aureus,* and *Klebsiella pneumoniae* was reported in 35% of spacers/VHCs used by children with asthma (109). Hence, it is recommended that patients should wash their spacers before first use and frequently thereafter (preferably weekly) according to the procedure outlined in Table 4.5. The spacer/VHC should not be washed in the dishwasher. Lukewarm tap water with a few drops of household detergent is recommended for cleaning (56). According to the manufacturer's instructions, the spacers/VHCs life is between 6 and 12 months and they should be replaced periodically, at least annually.

CONCLUSION

The appropriate use of spacers/VHCs to deliver pMDI aerosols can confer significant benefits for some patients, especially infants, children, the elderly, and those with acute exacerbations of asthma or COPD. The use of spacers/VHCs is more forgiving of errors related to actuation-inhalation incoordination. However, patients and clinicians need careful instructions about the nuances in correct use of spacers/VHCs to optimize treatment with these devices.

Table 4.5: **Washing and Cleaning Instructions for Spacers and VHCs**

- Disassemble the spacer/VHC after the last dose of the day
- Immerse in lukewarm water containing a few drops of household detergent
- Shake the parts in water and let it soak for 15 minutes
- Rinse the soapy water off the parts, including the mouthpiece with lukewarm water
- Do not rinse or rub the inside surfaces of the parts
- Place all the parts on a dry paper towel and air dry
- Reassemble the parts and ensure that the valve functions properly
- Wash the spacer/VHC frequently (preferably weekly)
- After each cleaning and drying and prior to use, prime the spacer/VHC by actuating 1 or 2 puffs from the pMDI into the spacer/VHC without inhaling the aerosol. Conducting metal spacers do not need priming
- Spacers should not be wrapped in a cloth for storage

Abbreviations: pMDI = pressurized metered-dose inhaler; VHC = valved holding chamber.

REFERENCES

1. Stein SW, Thiel CG. The history of therapeutic aerosols: A chronological review. J Aerosol Med Pulm Drug Deliv 2017;30:20–41. DOI:10.1089/jamp.2016.1297
2. Pritchard JN. The climate is changing for metered-dose inhalers and action is needed. Drug Des Devel Ther 2020;14:3043–3055.
3. Newman S. Respiratory drug delivery: The essential theory and practice. Richmond (VA): Respiratory Drug Delivery Online; 2009. p. 177–216. Chapter 6, Pressurized metered dose inhalers.
4. Kim CS, Eldridge A, Sackner MA. Oropharyngeal deposition and delivery aspects of metered-dose inhaler aerosols. Am Rev Respir Dis 1987;135:157–164.
5. Morén F. Drug deposition of pressurized inhalation aerosols I. Influence of actuator tube design. Int J Pharm 1978;1:205–212.
6. Newman SP, Millar AB, Lennard-Jones TR, et al. Pressurised aerosol deposition in the human lung with and without an "open" spacer device. Thorax 1989;44:706–710.
7. Corr D, Dolovich M, McCormack D, et al. Design and characteristics of a portable breath-actuated particle size selective medical aerosol inhaler. J Aerosol Sci 1982;13:1–7.
8. Newman SP, Millar AB, Lennard-Jones TR, et al. Improvement of pressurised aerosol deposition with Nebuhaler spacer device. Thorax 1984;39(12):935–941.
9. Epstein SW, Manning CPR, Ashley MJ, et al. Survey of the clinical use of pressurized aerosol inhalers. Can Med Assoc J 1979;120:813–816.
10. Dolovich M. Inhalation technique and inhalation devices. In: Pauwels R, O'Byrne P, editors. Lung biology in health and disease. New York (NY): Marcel Dekker, Inc.; 1997. p. 229–255. Chapter 10, Beta2-agonists in asthma treatment.
11. Liu X, Doub WH, Guo C. Evaluation of metered dose inhaler spray velocities using Phase Doppler Anemometry (PDA). Int J Pharm 2012;423:235–239.
12. Sarkar S, Peri SP, Chaudhury B. Investigation of multiphase multicomponent aerosol flow dictating pMDI-spacer interactions. Int J Pharm 2017;529:264–274.
13. Konig P. Spacer devices used with metered dose inhalers: Breakthrough or gimmick? Chest 1985;88:276–284.
14. Dalby RN, Somaraju S, Chavan VS, et al. Evaluation of aerosol drug output from the OptiChamber and AeroChamber spacers in a model system. J Asthma 1998;35:173–177.
15. Mitchell JP, Nagel MW, Rau JL. Performance of large-volume versus small-volume holding chambers with chlorofluorocarbon-albuterol and hydrofluoroalkane-albuterol sulfate. Respir Care 1999;44:38–44.
16. Salzman GA, Pyszczynski DR. Oropharyngeal candidiasis in patients treated with beclomethasone dipropionate delivered by metered-dose inhaler alone and with AeroChamber. J Allergy Clin Immunol 1988;81:424–428.
17. Newman SP, Moren F, Pavia D, et al. Deposition of pressurized suspension aerosol inhaled through extension devices. Am Rev Respir Dis 1981;124:317–320.
18. Roller CM, Zhang G, Troedsen RG, et al. Spacer inhalation technique and deposition of extrafine aerosol in asthmatic children. Eur Respir J 2007;29:299–306.

19. Dolovich MB. Influence of inspiratory flow rate, particle size, and airway caliber on aerosolized drug delivery to the lung. Respir Care 2000;45(6):597–608.

20. Lavorini F, Fontana GA. Targeting drugs to the airways: The role of spacer devices. Expert Opin Drug Deliv 2009;6:91–102.

21. Dolovich M, Ruffin R, Corr D, et al. Clinical evaluation of a simple demand inhalation MDI aerosol delivery device. Chest 1983;83(1):36–41.

22. Nikander K, Nicholls C, Denyer J, et al. The evolution of spacers and valved-holding chambers. J Aerosol Med Pulm Drug Deliv 2014;27:S4–S23.

23. Vincken W, Levy ML, Scullion J, et al. Spacer devices for inhaled therapy: Why use them and how? ERJ Open Res 2018;4:00065-2018. DOI:10.1183/23120541.00065-2018

24. O'Callaghan C, Barry P. Spacer devices in the treatment of asthma. BMJ 1997;314:1061.

25. Wilkes W, Fink J, Dhand R. Selecting an accessory device with a metered-dose inhaler: Variable influence of accessory devices on fine particle dose, throat deposition, and drug delivery with asynchronous actuation from a metered-dose inhaler. J Aerosol Med 2001;14(3):351–360.

26. Dolovich M. Lung dose, distribution, and clinical response to therapeutic aerosols. Aerosol Sci Technol 1993;18(3):230–240.

27. Dolovich M. Characterization of medical aerosols: Physical and clinical requirements for new inhalers. Aerosol Sci Technol 1995;22(4):392–399.

28. Finlay WH, Zuberbuhler P. In vitro comparison of salbutamol hydrofluoroalkane (Airomir) metered dose inhaler aerosols inhaled during pediatric tidal breathing from five valved holding chambers. J Aerosol Med 1999;12:285–291.

29. Nair A, Menzies D, Hopkinson P, et al. In vivo comparison of the relative systemic bioavailability of fluticasone propionate from three anti-static spacers and a metered dose inhaler. Br J Clin Pharmacol 2009;67:191–198.

30. Gillen M, Forte P, Svensson JO, et al. Effect of a spacer on total systemic and lung bioavailability in healthy volunteers and in vitro performance of the Symbicort® (budesonide/formoterol) pressurized metered dose inhaler. Pulm Pharmacol Ther 2018;52:7–17. DOI:10.1016/j.pupt.2018.08.001

31. Singh D, Collarini S, Poli G, et al. Effect of AeroChamber Plus™ on the lung and systemic bioavailability of beclometasone dipropionate/formoterol pMDI. Br J Clin Pharmacol 2011;72:932–939.

32. Dorinsky P, DePetrillo P, DeAngelis K, et al. Relative bioavailability of budesonide/glycopyrrolate/formoterol fumarate metered dose inhaler administered with and without a spacer: Results of a phase I, randomized, crossover trial in healthy adults. Clin Ther 2020;42(4):634–648. DOI:10.1016/j.clinthera.2020.02.012

33. O'Callaghan C, Lych J, Cant M, et al. Improvement in sodium cromoglycate delivery from a spacer device by use of an antistatic lining, immediate inhalation, and avoiding multiple actuation of drugs. Thorax 1993;46:603–606.

34. Clark DJ, Lipworth BJ. Effect of multiple actuations, delayed inhalation and antistatic treatment on the bioavailability of salbutamol via a spacer device. Thorax 1996;51:981–984.

35. Rau JL, Restrepo RD, Deshpande V. Inhalation of single vs multiple metered-dose bronchodilator actuations from reservoir devices: An in vitro study. Chest 1996;109:969–974.

36. Verbanck S, Vervaet C, Schuermans D, et al. Aerosol profile extracted from spacers as a determinant of actual dose. Pharm Res 2004;21(12):2213–2218. DOI:10.1007/s11095-004-7673-7.

37. Dubus JC, Dolovich M. Emitted doses of salbutamol pressurized metered-dose inhaler from five different plastic spacer devices. Fundam Clin Pharmacol 2000;14:219–224.

38. Holzner PM, Muller BW. An in vitro evaluation of various spacer devices for metered-dose inhalers using the Twin Impinger. Int J Pharm 1994;106:69–75.

39. Bisgaard H. Delivery of inhaled medication to children. J Asthma 1997;34(6):443–467.

40. Fink JB. Metered-dose inhalers, dry powder inhalers, and transitions. Respir Care 2000;45(6):623–635.

41. Ogrodnik N, Azzi V, Sprigge E, et al. Nonuniform deposition of pressurized metered-dose aerosol in spacer devices. J Aerosol Med Pulm Drug Deliv 2016;29:490–500.

42. Bisgaard H. A metal aerosol holding chamber devised for young children with asthma. Eur Respir J 1995;8(5):856–860.

43. Bisgaard H, Anhøj J, Klug B, et al. A non-electrostatic spacer for aerosol delivery. Arch Dis Child 1995;73(3):226–230.

44. Berg E, Madsen J, Bisgaard H. In vitro performance of three combinations of spacers and pressurized metered-dose inhalers for treatment of children. Eur Respir J 1998;12:472–476.

45. Kwok PCL, Chan H-K. Electrostatic charge in pharmaceutical systems. 2nd ed. New York (NY): Taylor & Francis Group, 2005. p. 1–14. (Encyclopedia of pharmaceutical technology).

46. Peart J, Magyar C, Byron PR. Aerosol electrostatics: Metered-dose inhalers (MDIs). In: Dalby RN, Byron PR, Farr SJ, editors. Respiratory drug delivery-VI. Buffalo Grove (IL): Interpharm Press; 1998. p. 227–233.

47. Glover W, Chan H-K. Electrostatic charge characterization of pharmaceutical aerosols using electrical low-pressure impaction (ELPI). J Aerosol Sci 2004;35(6):755–764.

48. Keil JC, Kotian R, Peart J. Using and interpreting aerosol electrostatic data from the electrical low pressure impactor. In: Dalby RN, Byron PR, Peart J, et al., editors. Respiratory drug delivery-X. River Grove (IL): Davis Horwood International Publishing; 2006. p. 267–277.

49. Bisgaard H, Anhoj J, Wildhaber JH. Spacer devices. In: Bisgaard H, O'Callaghan C, Smaldone GC, editors. Drug delivery to the lung. New York (NY): Marcel Dekker Inc.; 2002. p. 389–420.

50. Barry PW, O'Callaghan C. The effect of delay, multiple actuations and spacer static charge on the in vitro delivery of budesonide from the Nebuhaler. Br J Clin Pharmacol 1995;40:76–78.

51. Dewsbury NJ, Kenyon CJ, Newman SP. The effect of handling techniques on electrostatic charge on spacer devices: A correlation with in vitro particle size analysis. Int J Pharm 1996;137:261–264.

52. Kenyon CJ, Thorsson L, Borgstrom L, et al. The effects of static charge in spacer devices on glucocorticosteroid aerosol deposition in asthmatic patients. Eur Respir J 1998;11:606–610.

53. Peart J, Kulphaisal P, Orban JC. Relevance of electrostatics in respiratory drug delivery. Business Briefing: Pharmagenerics. 2003. Available from: http://www.touchbriefings.com/pdf/890/PT04_peart.pdf.

54. Janssens HM, Devadason SG, Hop WCJ, et al. Variability of aerosol delivery via spacer devices in young asthmatic children in daily life. Eur Respir J 1999;13:787–791.

55. Wildhaber JH, Devadason SG, Hayden MJ, et al. Electrostatic charge on plastic spacer devices influences the delivery of salbutamol. Eur Respir J 1996;9:1943–1946.

56. Pierart F, Wildhaber JH, Vrancken I, et al. Washing plastic spacers in household detergent reduces electrostatic charge and greatly improves delivery. Eur Respir J 1999;13:673–678.

57. Wildhaber JH, Devadason SG, Eber E, et al. Effect of electrostatic charge, flow, delay and multiple actuations on the in vitro delivery of salbutamol from different small volume spacers for infants. Thorax 1996;51(10):985–988.

58. Rau JL, Coppolo DP, Nagel MW, et al. The importance of nonelectrostatic materials in holding chambers for delivery of hydrofluoroalkane albuterol. Respir Care 2006;51(5):503–510.

59. Barry PW, O'Callaghan C. In vitro comparison of the amount of salbutamol available for inhalation from different formulations used with different spacer devices. Eur Respir J 1997;10(6):1345–1348. DOI:10.1183/09031936.9710061345

60. Dolovich M. Aerosols. In: Barnes PJ, Grunstein MM, Leff AR, et al., editors. Asthma. Philadelphia (NY): Lippincott-Raven; 1997. p. 1349–1366. Chapter 93.

61. Dolovich MB, Dhand R. Aerosol drug delivery: Developments in device design and clinical use. Lancet 2011;377(9770):1032–1045.

62. Levy ML, Hardwell A, McKnight E, et al. Asthma patients' inability to use a pressurised metered-dose inhaler (pMDI) correctly correlates with poor asthma control as defined by the global initiative for asthma (GINA) strategy: A retrospective analysis. Prim Care Respir J 2013;22:406–411.

63. Prabhakaran S, Shuster J, Chesrown S, et al. Response to albuterol MDI delivered through an anti-static chamber during nocturnal bronchospasm. Respir Care 2012;57(8):1291–1296.

64. Burudpakdee C, Kushnarev V, Coppolo D, et al. A retrospective study of the effectiveness of the AeroChamber Plus® Flow-Vu® antistatic valved holding chamber for asthma control. Pulm Ther 2017;3(2):283–296.

65. Ahrens R, Lux C, Bahl T, et al. Choosing the metered-dose inhaler spacer or holding chamber that matches the patient's need: Evidence that the specific drug being delivered is an important consideration. J Allergy and Clin Immunol 1995;96(2, Suppl 1):288–294.

66. Kenyon CJ, Dewsbury NJ, Newman SP. Differences in aerodynamic particle size distributions of innovator and generic beclomethasone dipropionate aerosols used with and without a large volume spacer. Thorax 1995;50:846–850.

67. Miller MR, Bright P. Differences in output from corticosteroid inhalers used with a volumatic spacer. Eur Respir J 1995;8:1637–1638.

68. Barry PW, O'Callaghan C. Inhalational drug delivery from seven different spacer devices. Thorax 1996;51:835–840.

69. Nagel MW, Wiersema KJ, Bates SL, et al. Performance of large- and small-volume valved holding chambers with a new combination long-term bronchodilator/anti-inflammatory formulation delivered by pressurized metered dose inhaler. J Aerosol Med 2002;15:427–433.

70. Lavorini F, Barreto C, van Boven JFM, et al. Spacers and valved holding chambers-the risk of switching to different chambers. J Allergy Clin Immunol Pract 2020;8(5):1569–1573.

71. Mitchell JP, Nagel MW. Valved holding chambers (VHCs) for use with pressurised metered-dose inhalers (pMDIs): A review of causes of inconsistent medication delivery. Prim Care Respir J 2007;16(4):207–214.

72. Williams RO III, Patel AM, Barron MK, et al. Investigation of some commercially available spacer devices for the delivery of glucocorticoid steroids from a pMDI. Drug Dev Ind Pharm 2001;27(5):401–412.

73. Dissanayake S, Nagel M, Falaschetti E, et al. Are valved holding chambers (VHCs) interchangeable? An in vitro evaluation of VHC equivalence. Pulm Pharmacol Ther 2018;48:179–184.

74. Childers AG, Cummings RH, Kaufman BD, et al. Comparative study of dose delivery and cascade impaction performance of four metered-dose inhaler and spacer combinations. Curr Ther Res 1996;57:75–87.

75. Brennan VK, Osman LM, Graham H, et al. True device compliance: The need to consider both competence and contrivance. Respir Med 2005;99:97–102.

76. Sanchis J, Gich I, Pedersen S. Aerosol Drug Management Improvement Team (ADMIT). Systematic review of errors in inhaler use: Has patient technique improved over time? Chest 2016;150(2):394–406. DOI:10.1016/j.chest.2016.03.041

77. Janssens HM, Tiddens HA. Aerosol therapy: The special needs of young children. Paediatr Respir Rev 2006;7(Suppl 1):S83–S85.

78. Newman SP, Pavia D, Garland N, et al. Effects of various inhalation modes on the deposition of radioactive pressurized aerosols. Eur J Respir Dis 1982;63(Suppl. 119):57–65.

79. Stephen D, Vatsa M, Lodha R, et al. A randomized controlled trial of 2 inhalation methods when using a pressurized metered dose inhaler with valved holding chamber. Respir Care 2015;60:1743–1748.

80. Berlinski A, von Hollen D, Hatley RHM, et al. Drug delivery in asthmatic children following coordinated and uncoordinated inhalation maneuvers: A randomized crossover trial. J Aerosol Med Pulm Drug Deliv 2017;30:182–189.

81. Janssens HM, Tiddens HAWM. Facemasks and aerosol delivery by metered dose inhaler-valved holding chamber in young children: A tight seal makes the difference. J Aerosol Med 2007;20(Suppl 1):S59–S65.

82. Smaldone GC, Sangwan S, Shah A. Facemask design, facial deposition, and delivered dose of nebulized aerosols. J Aerosol Med 2007;20(Suppl 1):S66–S77.

83. Shah SA, Berlinski AB, Rubin BK. Force-dependent static dead space of face masks used with holding chambers. Respir Care 2006;51(2):140–144.

84. Global Initiative for Asthma (GINA). 2022. [cited 2022 Jun 30]. Available from: https://ginasthma.org/wp-content/uploads/2022/05/GINA-Main-Report-2022-FINAL-22-05-03-WMS.pdf

85. UK National Institute for Clinical Excellence. Guidance on the use of inhaler systems(devices) in children under the age of 5 with chronic asthma. Technology Appraisal guidance No. 10 2000 [cited 2022 June 30]. Available from: http://www.nice.org.uk

86. Fitzgerald JM, Chan CK, Holroyde MC, et al. The CASE survey: Patient and physician perceptions regarding asthma medication use and associated oropharyngeal symptoms. Can Respir J 2008;15:27–32.

87. Hilton S. An audit of inhaler technique among asthma patients of 34 general practitioners. Br J Gen Pract 1990;40:505–506.

88. Guss D, Barash IA, Castillo EM. Characteristics of spacer device use by patients with asthma and COPD. J Emerg Med 2008;35:357–361.

89. Bryant L, Bang C, Chew C, et al. Adequacy of inhaler technique used by people with asthma or chronic obstructive pulmonary disease. J Prim Health Care 2013;5:191–198.

90. Pool JB, Greenough A, Gleeson JG, et al. Inhaled bronchodilator treatment via the Nebuhaler in young asthmatic patients. Arch Dis Child 1988;63:288–291.

91. Rau JL. Practical problems with aerosol therapy in COPD. Respir Care 2006;51:158–172.

92. Kerem E, Levison H, Schuh S, et al. Comparison with nebs in acute asthma in children. Efficacy of albuterol administered by nebulizer versus spacer device in children with acute asthma. J Pediatr 1993;123:313–317.

93. Parkin PC, Saunders NR, Diamond SA, et al. Randomized trial spacer vs. nebulizer for acute asthma. Arch Dis Child 1995;72:239–240.

94. Robertson CF, Norden MA, Fitzgerald DA, et al. Treatment of acute asthma: Salbutamol via jet nebulizer vs. spacer and metered dose inhaler. J Paediatr Child Health 1998;34:142–146.

95. Mandelberg A, Tsehori S, Houri S, et al. Is nebulized aerosol treatment necessary in the pediatric emergency department? Chest 2000;117:1309–1313.

96. Zar HJ, Streun S, Levin M, et al. Randomised controlled trial of the efficacy of a metered dose inhaler with bottle spacer for bronchodilator treatment in acute lower airway obstruction. Arch Dis Child 2007;92(2):142–146. DOI:10.1136/adc.2006.101642

97. Ho SF, OMahony MS, Steward JA, et al. Inhaler technique in older people in the community. Age Ageing 2004;33(2):185–188. DOI:10.1093/ageing/afh062

98. Lee H, Evans HE. Evaluation of inhalation aids of metered-dose inhalers in asthmatic children. Chest 1987;91:366–369.

99. Demirkan K, Tolley E, Mastin T, et al. Salmeterol administration by metered-dose inhaler alone vs metered-dose inhaler plus valved holding chamber. Chest 2000;117:1314–1318.

100. Lakamp RE, Berry TM, Prosser TR, et al. Compatibility of spacers with metered-dose inhalers. Am J Health Syst Pharm 2001;58(7):585–591.

101. Dolovich MB, Ahrens RC, Hess DR, et al. Device selection and outcomes of aerosol therapy: Evidence-based guidelines: American College of Chest Physicians/American College of Asthma, Allergy, and Immunology. Chest 2005;127(1):335–371.

102. Rodrigo C, Rodrigo G. Salbutamol treatment of acute severe asthma in the ED: MDI versus hand held nebulizer. Am J Emerg Med 1998;16:637–642.

103. Cates CJ, Welsh EJ, Rowe BH. Holding chambers (spacers) versus nebulisers for beta-agonist treatment of acute asthma. Cochrane Database Syst Rev 2013;9:CD000052.

104. van Geffen WH, Douma WR, Slebos DJ, et al. Bronchodilators delivered by nebuliser versus pMDI with spacer or DPI for exacerbations of COPD. Cochrane Database Syst Rev 2016;2016(8):CD011826. DOI:10.1002/14651858. CD011826.pub2

105. Idris AH, McDermott MF, Raucci JC, et al. Emergency department treatment of severe asthma. Metered-dose inhaler plus holding chamber is equivalent in effectiveness to nebulizer. Chest 1993;103:665–672.

106. Raimondi AC, Schottlender J, Lombardi D, et al. Treatment of acute severe asthma with inhaled albuterol delivered via jet nebulizer, metered dose inhaler with spacer, or dry powder. Chest 1997;112:24–28.
107. Slator L, von Hollen D, Sandell D, et al. In vitro comparison of the effect of inhalation delay and flow rate on the emitted dose from three valved holding chambers. J Aerosol Med Pulm Drug Deliv 2014;27(Suppl. 1):S37–S43.
108. Chambers FE, Brown S, Ludzik AJ. Comparative in vitro performance of valved holding chambers with a budesonide/formoterol pressurized metered-dose inhaler. Allergy Asthma Proc 2009;30(4):424–432. DOI:10.2500/aap.2009.30.3252
109. Cohen HA, Cohen Z, Pomeranz AS, et al. Bacterial contamination of spacer devices used by asthmatic children. J Asthma 2005;42:169–172.

5 Slow Mist Inhalers

P. N. Richard Dekhuijzen, Matteo Bonini, and Federico Lavorini

CONTENTS

INTRODUCTION

Slow mist inhalers (SMIs) have been part of the spectrum of inhalation devices since 2003. They are considered to be a separate class of inhaler devices, besides pMDIs, DPIs, and nebulizers.

WHAT IS AN SMI?

In essence, the SMI is classified as a pocket-sized device that can generate a single-breath aerosol from a propellant-free liquid drug solution (1). SMIs deliver the drug solution using mechanical energy produced by a spring, generating a fine, slow-moving mist over a longer period compared to other devices (1.2–1.5 s versus 0.15–0.35 s). This allows patients more time to synchronize actuation and breathing, possibly reducing the errors due to poor coordination. The slow-moving mist also reduces the requirements for a high inspiratory effort by the patient. Of relevance, SMIs offer advanced technology containing a high small-particle fraction, resulting in low drug deposition in the oropharynx and high total lung deposition (>50%), effectively targeting the site of disease (2). However, patients using SMIs may require additional support in the assembly and proper priming procedures (3). Like pMDIs, SMIs can also be combined with spacers, although the combination is yet to be fully evaluated. In addition, the Respimat inhaler with a T-piece adapter can be safely used to deliver medications in mechanically ventilated tracheostomized patients (4).

The only SMI currently available is the Soft Mist Inhaler Respimat, developed by Boehringer Ingelheim. This device contains different bronchodilators as separate entities and in combinations. Other SMIs are in development, e.g., by Merxin (5).

DOI: 10.1201/9781003269014-5

HOW DOES A SMI WORK?

The Respimat SMI uses a nozzle system (the Uniblock) to aerosolize a metered dose of drug solution into tiny particles suitable for inhalation (6). A schematic overview of the Respimat and its components is shown in Figure 5.1 (7). The Respimat SMI generates an aerosol independently of the patient's inhalation effort, with a slow velocity and prolonged duration, which may facilitate the coordination of actuation and inhalation. Since the aerosol generated by the Respimat SMI has a high fine-particle fraction delivered at a slow velocity, lung deposition is maximized and

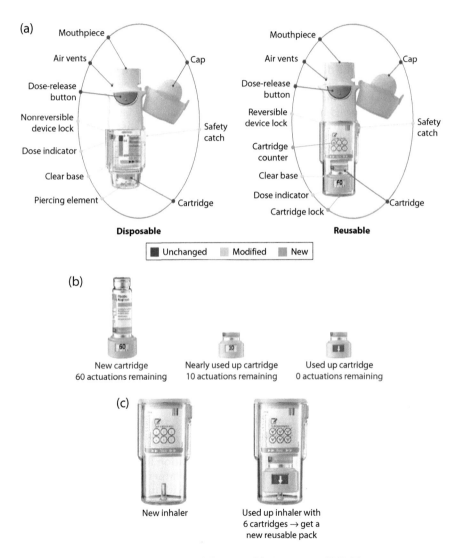

Figure 5.1 Schematic drawing of the reusable Respimat SMI (7).

oropharyngeal deposition minimized, even at low inhalation flows. More than 60% of the drug dose released by the Respimat SMI falls within a fine-particle dose of <5.0 μm, which enhances drug delivery to the smaller bronchi and bronchioles (8).

The Respimat SMI has a favorable lung deposition profile in patients with asthma or COPD. In six patients with asthma, drug deposition to the whole lung and the peripheral airways using the Respimat SMI (57.1% and 39.7%, respectively) was higher than when using MDIs or DPIs (whole lung deposition 20.0–44.3%; peripheral airway deposition 11.3–29.2%). The deposition fractions for the Respimat SMI in the upper, central, and peripheral airways were in the ranges of 41.3–44.3%, 13.8–22.6%, and 34.6–42.4%, respectively (8).

Mechanisms to release drug differ significantly among inhaler types. Patients have to generate a certain inspiratory flow through DPIs to disperse the drug and get it out of the device and into the lungs. So, users have to generate a certain inspiratory flow rate to overcome the resistance in the DPI. In case of high internal resistance, patients have to generate a sharp and fast (2–3 seconds) inspiration, followed by a breath hold of 5–10 seconds (the latter is the case for all inhaler types). In case of lower internal resistance, the inspiration through the device may be less powerful. In case of a pMDI, the drug is released after actuation of the device, irrespective of the inspiratory flow. Clearly, however, there must be an inspiratory maneuver in order to get the released drug into the airways. The inspiratory flow through the SMI, however, may be low, e.g., 30 liters/min. The release of drugs from an SMI is initiated by actuating the device. Again, lung deposition occurs only when the patient inhales simultaneously, but the inhalation may be at low flow rates as with pMDIs. A significant advantage of the SMI is the low plume velocity which enables the patient to inhale the dose even more easily. In vivo studies have confirmed that lung deposition after inhaling through an SMI of pMDI is higher than through a DPI (9).

This improved deposition in the lungs combined with reduced oropharyngeal deposition is caused by the slower aerosol velocity of the Respimat SMI relative to other inhalers. The aerosol spray velocity of the Respimat SMI (0.84 and 0.72 m/s at 80 and 100 mm from the end of the nozzle, respectively) is lower than that of seven different pMDIs; the slowest MpDI spray velocity was 2.47 and 1.71 m/s at 80 and 100 mm from the end of the nozzle, respectively (10). Similarly, the Respimat SMI produces an aerosol cloud that moves much more slowly than aerosol clouds from pMDIs (mean velocity 100 mm from the nozzle: Respimat SMI, 0.8 m/s; MDIs, 2.0–8.4 m/s). The soft mist produced by the Respimat SMI had a longer mean duration (1.5 s) than that produced by MDIs (0.15–0.36 s) (11).

Recently, an improved second-generation Respimat reusable inhaler was released. In more detail, this second-generation Respimat inhaler is characterized by an easier device assembly, a larger dose indicator window, and, more importantly, it is reusable, with up to six cartridges with an intuitive cartridge-exchange mechanism (7). The updated design was intended to improve the usability and environmental impact of the Respimat inhaler while preserving the pharmaceutical performance and basic functions of the disposable Respimat inhaler. The reusable version of the Respimat has improved usability, with no effect on the efficiency of drug delivery, aerosol particle size, or required inhalation method across multiple cartridge use. Furthermore, studies assessing patients' satisfaction and preferences indicate that the new reusable version of Respimat has consistently been shown to be well accepted by patients with asthma and COPD with a high degree of patients' satisfaction.

There could also be potential environmental benefits of reusable inhalers. The carbon footprint of an item, individual, or organization, is one of the most important and quantifiable environmental impacts, assessed by the amount of greenhouse gases (often expressed in terms of CO_2 equivalents) generated throughout the lifecycle. At variance with pMDIs that contain hydrofluorocarbon (HFC) propellants (HFC-134a and HFC-227ea), which are potent greenhouse gases, SMIs such as the Respimat do not require propellants since the energy to dispense an aqueous solution as a mist of particles is provided by a spring. Hänsel et al. compared the carbon footprints of Respimat versus pMDIs for several drug combinations, including Respimat reusable and disposable (12). They found that switching from an HFC pMDI to a disposable Respimat resulted in an approximate 95% reduction in the lifecycle carbon footprint. Compared with the disposable device over one month, use of the Respimat reusable over three months would further reduce the monthly carbon footprint to 0.34 kg CO_2 eq (corresponding to a 57% reduction), or 0.23 kg CO_2 eq if used over 6 months (a 71% reduction).

WHICH MEDICATIONS ARE AVAILABLE IN AN SMI?

The Respimat SMI device contains different bronchodilators (Table 5.1): short-acting beta-2-agonists (fenoterol), ultralong-acting beta-2-agonists (olodaterol), short-acting anticholinergics (ipratropium bromide), two combinations of a short-acting anticholinergic and a short-acting beta-2-agonist (ipratropium plus salbutamol, and ipratropium plus fenoterol), ultralong-acting anticholinergics (tiotropium), and the combination of an ultralong-acting anticholinergic and an ultralong-acting beta-2-agonist (tiotropium plus olodaterol). Inhaled corticosteroids are not available in this device.

HOW SHOULD SMIs BE USED?

The instructions on how to use an SMI are available in several languages. The English version is available at https://www.medical.respimat.com/ie/HCP/how-to-use#:~:text=Point%20the%20inhaler%20to%20the%20back%20of%20the,10%20seconds%20or%20for%20as%20long%20as%20comfortable (13).

For daily use, there are three steps: turn, open, and press.

Table 5.1: Medications Available in SMIs

Short-acting beta-2-agonists	Fenoterol
Ultralong-acting beta-2-agonists	Olodaterol
Short-acting anticholinergics	Ipratropium bromide
Short-acting anticholinergic combined with a short-acting beta-2-agonist	Ipratropium plus salbutamol Ipratropium plus fenoterol
Ultralong-acting anticholinergics	Tiotropium
Ultralong-acting anticholinergic combined with an ultralong-acting beta-2-agonist	Tiotropium plus olodaterol

Abbreviation: SMI = slow mist inhalers.

51

TURN

- Keep the cap closed.
- **TURN** the clear base in the direction of the arrows on the label until it clicks (half a turn).

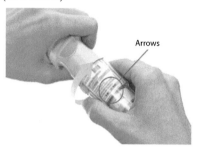

Arrows

OPEN

- **OPEN** the cap until it snaps fully open.

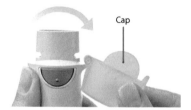

Cap

PRESS

- Breathe out slowly and fully.
- Close the lips around the mouthpiece without covering the air vents. Point the inhaler to the back of the throat.
- While taking a slow, deep breath through the mouth, **PRESS** the dose-release button and continue to breathe in slowly for as long as comfortable.
- Hold the breath for 10 seconds or for as long as comfortable.
- Repeat **TURN, OPEN, PRESS** for a total of 2 puffs.
- Close the cap until the inhaler is used again.

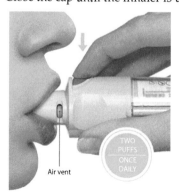

Air vent

IS THE SMI USED AS RESCUE THERAPY?

The SMIs containing short-acting beta-2-agonists and/or short-acting anticholinergics can be used as rescue therapy.

IS THE SMI USED AS MAINTENANCE THERAPY?

The SMIs containing long-acting beta-2-agonists and/or long-acting anticholinergics can be used as maintenance therapy.

ADVANTAGES OF SMIs FOR PATIENTS AND HCPs

Several studies and reviews have shown that poor inhalation technique may severely impact the clinical efficacy of medications, resulting in impaired disease control, worsening quality of life, increased exacerbation and mortality risk, increased hospitalization, and, in turn, increased health care expenditure. Factors like ease of use will influence actual use, patient preferences, and adherence (1, 14, 15).

Some characteristics of the Respimat device may support its ease of use. Patients only need to generate a low inspiratory flow rate through the device to get the medication into the airways. The low velocity of the plume and the long plume duration enable the patient to inhale an optimal portion of the delivered dose. And finally, the high fine-particle fraction ensures a high deposition throughout the entire lung. Patients may appreciate the lack of propellants that might contribute to the carbon footprint, and the availability of a reusable device (up to five times, by replacing an empty canister with a new one) (1).

Patients may rank their experiences and appreciation of an inhaler using the Patient Satisfaction and Preference Questionnaire (PASAPQ). The Respimat SMI scored high in the performance and convenience domains (16).

In a comparative analysis of adherence with seven different types of inhalers, the Respimat SMI was associated with the lowest risk of underuse (5.5%), defined as taking < 50% of the doses prescribed, in patients with COPD (1). MDIs were associated with a higher rate of overuse (taking > 125% of doses) and a lower rate of optimal use (= 75% and = 125%) compared with Respimat SMI in this analysis (17).

Comparative studies have been performed with SMIs, pMDIs, and DPIs. Comparing SMIs and pMDIs, patients (n = 201) significantly favored the Respimat SMI, with 81% reporting a preference for Respimat SMI compared to a pMDI (18). Compared to DPIs, the total satisfaction score in 153 patients with asthma was higher for the Respimat SMI (85.5) than for DPI (76.9), and the majority of patients preferred the Respimat SMI (74%) to DPI (17%) (19).

DISADVANTAGES OF SMIs FOR PATIENTS AND HCPs

Possible disadvantages of the Respimat SMI are that the device needs some basic assembly and priming before the first use. Some patients, especially those with manual dexterity impairment, may have difficulty putting the cartridge into the base, following the Turn-Open-Press procedure, and then priming the device. Children may also find it difficult to produce adequate airflow to correctly operate some inhalers. In a study in children (aged < 5 years) with respiratory disease, 83% of 4-year-olds achieved adequate inhalation using the Respimat SMI unaided or with parental help, and 100% of 3- to 4-year-olds achieved adequate inhalation with the addition of a valved holding chamber (20). Another disadvantage of the currently available SMIs is that they do not contain ICS, either as a single agent or in combination with a long-acting beta-2-agonist or together with a beta-2-agonist and a long-acting anticholinergic.

COMMON ERRORS WHEN USING SMIs

In a recent meta-analysis, the mistakes when using an SMI, as reported in eleven studies, were analyzed (21). Among the eleven studies with step-by-step data, the most common errors were failure to (1) exhale completely and away from the device (47.8% (95% CI: 33.6–62.0)); (2) hold the breath for up to 10 seconds (30.6% (95% CI: 17.5–43.7)); (3) take a slow, deep breath while pressing the dose-release button (27.9% (95% CI: 14.5–41.2)); (4) hold the inhaler upright (22.6% (95% CI: 6.2–39.0)); and (5) turn the base toward the arrows until it clicked (17.6% (95% CI: 3.0–32.2)). Device use errors occurred in about 6 of 10 patients who used SMIs. Data on errors after addressing these issues by repeated training are not available to the best of our knowledge.

CONCLUSIONS

The currently available SMI (Respimat) has a number of features that may support patients in its correct use. These characteristics include the low inspiratory flow needed to inhale the drug properly, the low velocity and long plume duration, and the high fine-particle fraction. In clinical studies, these features appear to translate into a positive appreciation of its ease of use.

REFERENCES

1. Iwanaga T, Tohda Y, Nakamura S, Suga Y. The Respimat Soft Mist Inhaler: implications of drug delivery characteristics for patients. Clin Drug Investig 2019;39:1021–1030.
2. Bonini M, Usmani OS. Demystifying inhaler use in chronic obstructive airways disease. Barc Respir Netw Rev 2018;4(4):304–318.
3. Baiardini I, Braido F, Bonini M, et al. Why do doctors and patients not follow guidelines? Curr Opin Allergy Clin Immunol 2009;9:228–233.
4. Mehri R, Alatrash A, Ogrodnik N, et al. In vitro measurements of Spiriva Respimat dose delivery in mechanically ventilated tracheostomy patients. J Aerosol Med Pulm Drug Deliv 2021;34:242–250.
5. MRX004. [cited 2022 Mar 26]. Available from: https://www.merxin.com/products/mrx004
6. Wachtel H, Kattenbeck S, Dunne S, et al. The Respimat development story: Patient-centered innovation. Pulm Ther 2017;3:19–30.
7. Dhand R, Eicher J, Hänsel M, et al. Improving usability and maintaining performance: Human-factor and aerosol-performance studies evaluating the new reusable Respimat inhaler. Int J Chron Obstruct Pulmon Dis 2019;14:509–523.
8. Perriello EA, Sobieraj DM. The Respimat Soft Mist Inhaler, a novel inhaled drug delivery device. Conn Med 2016;80:359–364.
9. Iwanaga T, Kozuka T, Nakanishi J, et al. Aerosol deposition of inhaled corticosteroids/long-acting β_2-agonists in the peripheral airways of patients with asthma using functional respiratory imaging, a novel imaging technology. Pulm Ther 2017;3:219–231.
10. Hochrainer D, Holz H, Kreher C, et al. Comparison of the aerosol velocity and spray duration of Respimat Soft Mist inhaler and pressurized metered dose inhalers. J Aerosol Med 2005;18:273–282.
11. Tamura G. Comparison of the aerosol velocity of Respimat Soft Mist inhaler and seven pressurized metered dose inhalers. Allergol Int 2015;64:390–392.

12. Hänsel M, Bambach T, Wachtel H. Reduced environmental impact of the reusable Respimat® Soft Mist™ Inhaler compared with pressurised metered-dose Inhalers. Adv Ther 2019;36:2487–2492.

13. How to use the Respimat device. [cited 2022 Mar 26]. Available from: https://www.medical.respimat.com/ie/HCP/how-to-use#:~:text=Point%20 the%20inhaler%20to%20the%20back%20of%20the,10%20seconds%20or%20 for%20as%20long%20as%20comfortable

14. Bourbeau J, Bartlett SJ. Patient adherence in COPD. Thorax 2008;63:831–838.

15. Small M, Anderson P, Vickers A, et al. Importance of inhaler-device satisfaction in asthma treatment: Real-world observations of physician-observed compliance and clinical/patient reported outcomes. Adv Ther 2011;28:202–212.

16. Davis KH, Su J, González JM, et al. Quantifying the importance of inhaler attributes corresponding to items in the patient satisfaction and preference questionnaire in patients using Combivent Respimat. Health Qual Life Outcomes 2017;15:201.

17. Koehorst-ter Huurne K, Movig K, van der Valk P, et al. The influence of type of inhalation device on adherence of COPD patients to inhaled medication. Expert Opin Drug Deliv 2016;13:469–475.

18. Schurmann W, Schmidtmann S, Moroni P, et al. Respimat Soft Mist inhaler versus hydrofluoroalkane metered dose inhaler: Patient preference and satisfaction. Treat Respir Med 2005;4:53–61.

19. Hodder R, Reese PR, Slaton T. Asthma patients prefer Respimat® Soft Mist™ Inhaler to Turbuhaler. Int J Chron Obstruct Pulmon Dis 2009;4:225–232.

20. Kamin W, Frank M, Kattenbeck S, et al. A handling study to assess use of the Respimat Soft Mist Inhaler in children under 5 years old. J Aerosol Med Pulm Drug Deliv 2015;28:372–381.

21. Navaie M, Dembek C, Cho-Reyes S, et al. Device errors with soft mist inhalers: A global systematic review and meta-analysis. Chronic Respir Dis 2020;17:1–13.

6 Dry Powder Inhalers

Donald A. Mahler and Roy A. Pleasants

CONTENTS

WHAT IS A DRY POWDER INHALER?

A dry powder inhaler (DPI) is a hand-held device that contains a powder medication that can be inhaled by an individual into the lower respiratory tract. The first DPI introduced was Intal Spinhaler® (sodium cromoglycate) by Fisons in the United Kingdom in 1967 and in the United States in 1970, to prevent both immediate and late antigen-induced asthmatic reactions (1). The developers found that sodium cromoglycate needed to be attached to lactose as a carrier particle to achieve effective delivery of the medication with the Spinhaler®, a feature that remains a critical aspect of DPI formulation (1). The next DPI introduced was the Rotohaler® in 1977 by Allen & Hanburys for the delivery of albuterol (1).

Although the Spinhaler® and Rotohaler® are relatively inefficient devices for drug delivery to the lung, the development process provided a background for the subsequent proliferation of DPIs following the signing of the Montreal Protocol in 1987 (see Chapter 1). The intent of his global agreement was to protect the ozone layer by phasing out the production and consumption of ozone-depleting substances such as chlorofluorocarbons (CFCs) which were used as a propellant in pressurized metered-dose inhalers (pMDI) (2).

There are three basic types of DPIs (Figure 6.1). 1) A single-unit device in which a capsule is inserted into a cavity within the DPI and is then punctured by a piercing apparatus before dosing; Aerolizer®, Breezhaler®, and HandiHaler® are examples. 2) A multi-unit device which contains a number or series of blisters; as found in the Accuhaler®/Diskus®, Ellipta®, and Genuair®/Pressair® DPIs. 3) A reservoir device which contains a bulk amount of drug powder with an internal mechanism to provide/deliver a single dose upon actuation. Examples of reservoir DPI are the Digihaler®, Easyhaler®, and Turbohaler®/Turbuhaler® (3).

Most DPIs are dispensed in sealed foil packaging with a desiccant to protect the drug formulation from environmental moisture. Both high humidity as well as the patient's exhalation into the mouthpiece of the DPI can reduce the amount of respirable drug emitted, due to the clumping of the powder and consequently

DOI: 10.1201/9781003269014-6

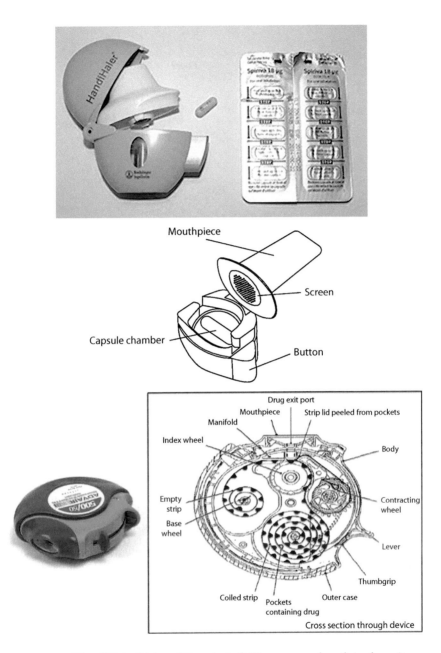

Figure 6.1 HandiHaler® (a) and Breezhaler® (b) are examples of single-unit devices in which a capsule is inserted into a cavity. (c) The Diskus® is a multi-unit-dose dry powder inhaler that contains a number of blisters. Internal components of the Diskus® are shown on the right. (d) The Turbuhaler® is a reservoir dry powder inhaler that contains a bulk amount of drug powder with an internal mechanism to deliver a single dose upon actuation.

(*Continued*)

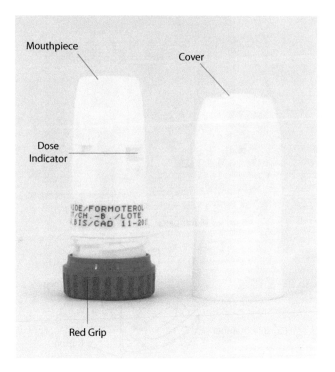

Mouthpiece

Cover

Dose
Indicator

DE/FORMOTEROL
/CH.-B./LOTE
BIS/CAD 11-20

Red Grip

Figure 6.1 (*Continued*)

reduced dispersal of fine particles (4). DPIs should be stored in a dry location with average relative humidity below 40–45% (5).

HOW DOES A DPI WORK?

Most dry powder formulations consist of a mixture of micronized drug less than five microns (μm) in mass median aerodynamic diameter attached to larger carrier particles (usually lactose) which act as bulking agents and improve the flowability of the powder. An alternative formulation is that of micronized drug particles as agglomerates in a packet or pellet. DPIs are activated when the patient inhales through the device, creating turbulent energy that aerosolizes, disaggregates, and disperses the powder formulation into respirable particles (3) (Figure 6.2). As the drug leaves the metering cup inside the DPI during the first few milliseconds, the beginning of inhalation should be "fast." If this does not occur, drug particles remain too large and are deposited in the mouth (6).

Peak Inspiratory Flow

The generation of turbulent energy within DPIs is determined by the individual's peak inspiratory flow (PIF) and the internal resistance (r) of the DPI (3) (Table 6.1). The PIFr can be measured using an inspiratory flow meter and is defined as the maximum airflow generated during inhalation through the simulated resistance of a DPI (7). In vitro studies using lung models have established both minimal and optimal PIF values that have been extrapolated for clinical application (8–10).

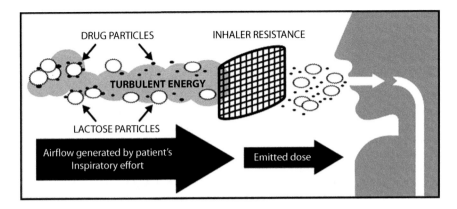

Figure 6.2 For most dry powder formulations, the drug particles are attached to a lactose carrier which acts as a bulking agent and improves the flowability of the powder. By inhaling through the device, the patient creates turbulent energy that disaggregates and disperses the powder formulation into respirable particles. Turbulent energy is determined by the patient's peak inspiratory flow and the internal resistance of the dry powder inhaler (DPI).

Minimal PIFr

A minimal PIFr is required for each DPI to *initiate* disaggregation of the powder, with 30 liters/minute recommended for low-to-medium high-resistance DPIs and 20 liters/minute for high-resistance DPIs (10, 12). If PIFr is below this minimal value, disaggregation of the powder formulation is ineffective. This leads to a reduced fine-particle dose emitted from the device and results in the patient receiving little or no therapeutic effect (3).

Optimal PIFr

In vitro studies using lung models show that drug delivery and the fine-particle dose (< 5 μm in diameter) are enhanced with increasing inspiratory flows (8, 9). An optimal PIFr is determined when a plateau occurs in the emitted dose and fine-particle dose despite higher inspiratory flows (8). There is a general

Table 6.1: Dry Powder Inhalers According to Their Internal Resistance

Internal Resistance	Dry Powder Inhaler
Low	Breezhaler®
Medium–low	Accuhaler®/Diskus®, Diskhaler®, and Ellipta®
Medium	Clickhaler®, Genuair®/Pressair®, InHub®, Digihaler®/RespiClick®/Spiromax® and Turbuhaler® (Symbicort)
Medium–high	Easyhaler® (combination), Flexhaler®/Turbohaler®/Turbuhaler® (Pulmicort), NEXThaler®, and Twisthaler®
High	Easyhaler® (monotherapy) and HandiHaler®

Note: Dry powder inhalers are listed in alphabetical order within the five resistance groupings according to Clerk Clement International Limited (7). For InHub, the airflow resistance is 0.035 kPa$^{0.5}$ liters/minute, placing it in the medium-resistance category (11).

consensus that an optimal PIFr $\geq$ 60 liters/minute applies to most low-to-medium high-resistance DPIs and $\geq$ 30 liters/minute for high-resistance DPIs (3, 12, 13). Moreover, PIFr can be considered a predictive therapeutic biomarker to assess whether an individual patient is unlikely to achieve optimal drug delivery and clinical benefit when using a DPI (14).

WHAT DRY POWDER INHALERS AND MEDICATIONS ARE AVAILABLE?

Dry powder inhaler devices and medications approved for the treatment of asthma and/or COPD are listed in Table 6.2. All classes of dry powder devices/medications are available except for short-acting muscarinic antagonist (SAMA) bronchodilators. These include short- (SABA) and long-acting beta-agonist (LABA) bronchodilators, long-acting muscarinic antagonist (LAMA) bronchodilators, inhaled corticosteroids (ICS), LABA/LAMA combinations, ICS/LABA combinations, and an ICS/LABA/LAMA combination.

HOW SHOULD A DPI BE USED?

In general, information for a DPI ("Instructions for Use" in the United States and "Patient Information Leaflet" in Europe) describes that after preparing the inhaler device (e.g., pressing the lever or opening the cover and placing the capsule in the device), the patient should hold the inhaler away from the mouth and then breathe out completely, making sure not to exhale directly into the mouthpiece. The individual then inserts the mouthpiece into the mouth and closes the lips. Inhalation instructions are provided by each pharmaceutical company and are different for each DPI (15).

In 2009, Magnussen et al. (16) examined the effects of two different inhalation instructions on PIF measured through the HandiHaler® device. These investigators found that PIF was approximately 13 liters/minute higher when patients with COPD performed a "fast, forceful" inhalation compared with a "slow, deep" effort (16). In 2011, a joint task force of the European Respiratory Society and the International Society for Aerosols in Medicine provided recommendations for patients to inhale "forcefully from the beginning of inhalation" when using a DPI (3). A simple instruction for patients is to inhale "hard and fast" (17). For DPIs that contain capsules, it is recommended that patients repeat the inhalation to ensure receiving the full dose (3). After complete inhalation, the patient should hold the breath for "as long as possible" or for up to 10 seconds to enable the fine particles to deposit deep into the lower respiratory tract (3).

Mechanical and electromechanical devices have been developed for DPIs to help guide patients to achieve adequate inhalations. The In Check DIAL® is a portable inspiratory flow meter that has been used to measure PIFr to assess whether the patient can generate optimal turbulent energy within the DPI (7). Two specific DPIs incorporate a mechanism that requires a threshold inspiratory flow to allow the release of the powder medication from the device. Genuair®/Pressair® (AstraZeneca, Wilmington, DE) is a medium-resistance DPI that requires a minimum inspiratory flow of 40 liters/minute to allow the trigger mechanism to provide acoustic and optical signals that the individual patient has inhaled the medication successfully (16, 18). The NEXThaler® (Chiesi, Parma, Italy) is a medium-high-resistance DPI with a breath actuation mechanism that limits dose release until the pressure drop across the device is approximately 1.8 kPa (19). This guarantees that the dose is released only when the individual achieves a threshold inspiratory flow of at least 35 liters/minute (19). In addition, DPIs can have built-in (Teva Digihaler®) or attachable (Hailie®,

Table 6.2: Dry Powder Inhaler Devices and Medications Approved for the Treatment of Asthma and/or COPD

Inhaler Device	Medication (Generic)	Frequency of Use
	Short-acting beta-agonist	
Clickhaler	Albuterol	4–6 hours PRN[a]
Digihaler/RespiClick/ Spiromax	Albuterol	4–6 hours PRN[a]
Turbuhaler	Terbutaline	4–6 hours PRN[a]
	Long-acting beta-agonist (LABA)	
Accuhaler/Diskus	Salmeterol	Twice daily
Breezhaler	Indacaterol	Once daily
Diskhaler	Salmeterol	Twice daily
	Long-acting muscarinic antagonist (LAMA)	
Breezhaler	Glycopyrronium	Once daily
Ellipta	Umeclidinium	Once daily
Genuair/Pressair	Aclidinium	Twice daily
HandiHaler	Tiotropium	Once daily
	Inhaled corticosteroid (ICS)	
Clickhaler	Budesonide	Twice daily
Digihaler/RespiClick/ Spiromax	Fluticasone propionate	Twice daily
Easyhaler	Budesonide	Twice daily
Flexhaler/Turbuhaler	Budesonide	Twice daily
Twisthaler	Mometasone furoate	Twice daily
	LABA/LAMA	
Breezhaler	Indacaterol and glycopyrronium	Once daily
Ellipta	Vilanterol and umeclidinium	Once daily
Genuair/Pressair	Formoterol and aclidinium	Twice daily
	ICS/LABA	
Accuhaler/Diskus	Fluticasone propionate and salmeterol	Twice daily
Digihaler/RespiClick/ Spiromax	Fluticasone propionate and salmeterol	Twice daily
Easyhaler	Fluticasone propionate and salmeterol	Twice daily
Ellipta	Fluticasone furoate and vilanterol	Once daily
InHub	Fluticasone propionate and salmeterol	Twice daily
NEXThaler	Beclomethasone and formoterol	Twice daily
Turbuhaler	Budesonide and formoterol	Twice daily
	ICS/LABA/LAMA	
Ellipta	Fluticasone furoate, vilanterol, and umeclidinium	Once daily

[a] Pro re nata or as needed.

Adherium Ltd, Auckland, New Zealand) sensors that measure inspiratory flow along with inspiratory volume and provide digital information/feedback.

IS A DPI USED AS RELIEVER/RESCUE THERAPY?

Both albuterol and terbutaline are available in DPIs that can be used "as needed" to relieve symptoms in those with asthma and COPD (Table 6.2). However, since 2019, the Global Initiative for Asthma (GINA) has recommended against SABA-only treatment of asthma, as the use of one or more SABA canisters per month is associated with an increased risk of exacerbations and mortality (20). To control symptoms and to reduce the risk of serious exacerbations, GINA recommends that "All adults and adolescents with asthma should be treated with ICS-containing therapy: either regularly every day or, in mild asthma, with ICS-formoterol taken as needed for symptom relief" (21).

The 2021 GINA strategy proposed two treatment tracks for asthma (21). For *Track 1*, low-dose ICS-formoterol is recommended as a reliever because it reduces the risk of severe exacerbations compared with using a SABA reliever with/without a maintenance controller (21). Both beclomethasone-formoterol (NEXThaler®) and budesonide-formoterol (Turbuhaler®) are the available DPIs for such use (Table 6.2). For *Track 2*, SABA as the reliever is proposed as an alternative approach along with daily ICS maintenance therapy (21).

For COPD, the 2022 Global Initiative for Obstructive Lung Disease (GOLD) recommends that "Rescue short-acting bronchodilators should be prescribed for all patients for immediate symptom relief" (22). For initial pharmacotherapy for patients with low symptoms and a low risk of exacerbations (Group A), the GOLD strategy proposes either a short-acting or a long-acting bronchodilator (22).

IS A DPI USED AS MAINTENANCE THERAPY?

DPIs are used widely, as once- or twice-daily maintenance therapy, for patients with asthma and COPD. For patients with asthma, GINA has recommended that patients take ICS-formoterol as daily maintenance treatment and as needed for symptom relief in steps 3–5 of *Track 1* (21). Both beclomethasone-formoterol (NEXThaler®) and budesonide-formoterol (Turbuhaler®) are available DPIs for maintenance and reliever therapy, respectively (Table 6.2). For *Track 2*, step 2, low-dose maintenance ICS therapy is recommended by GINA, of which budesonide (Clickhaler®, Easyhaler®, Flexhaler®/Turbuhaler®), fluticasone propionate (Digihaler®/RespiClick®/Spiromax®), and mometasone furoate (Twisthaler®) are available (21) (Table 6.2). For steps 3–5 in *Track 2*, ICS-LABA maintenance treatment is recommended with beclomethasone-formoterol (NEXThaler®) and budesonide-formoterol (Turbuhaler®), available as DPIs (Table 6.2). For step 5 in both *Tracks 1 and 2*, add-on LAMA therapy has been proposed by GINA (21). Available dry powder LAMAs include Breezhaler®, Ellipta®, Genuair®/Pressair®, and HandiHaler® devices (Table 6.2).

For patients with COPD, monotherapy with LABA or LAMA as well as a combination LABA/LAMA has been recommended for the treatment of symptomatic patients (22–25). The DPI options for this COPD phenotype include three LABAs, four LAMAs, and three LABA/LAMA combination bronchodilators (Table 6.2). The ICS/LABA and ICS/LABA/LAMA combinations have been recommended for patients who have high symptoms and/or are considered at increased risk for an exacerbation (22, 23, 25). Seven ICS/LABA combination DPIs are available, while there is one ICS/LABA/LAMA dry powder inhaler (Ellipta®) (Table 6.2). Furthermore, Bourbeau et al. (24) have suggested ICS/LABA/LAMA "triple therapy" for patients with persistent dyspnea and poor health status.

ADVANTAGES OF A DPI

For Patients

A major advantage for patients is that DPIs are breath-actuated such that hand-breath coordination is not required. In contrast, actuation of a pMDI (i.e., press down on the canister) and a slow mist inhaler (SMI) (i.e., press a button) needs to be coordinated with inhalation for optimal deposition of the medication into the lower respiratory tract (see Chapters 3 and 5).

For Patients and HCPs

As noted in Table 6.2, two or more different medications and/or combinations are available in the same DPI: Accuhaler®/Diskus®, Breezhaler®, Digihaler®/RespiClick®/Spiromax®, Easyhaler®, Ellipta®, Genuair®/Pressair®, and Turbohaler®/Turbuhaler®. This availability provides inhaler familiarity and continuity for both patients and HCPs, making it easier to "step up" or "step down" therapy. Moreover, HCPs can instruct patients on the same exhalation/inhalation technique for using a particular DPI after the device has been prepared.

For the Environment

DPIs do not contain a propellant, and their minimal carbon footprint is mainly attributed to raw materials and manufacturing. Although hydrofluoroalkanes were developed as an alternative propellant for pMDIs, they are greenhouse gases and are planned to be phased down under the Kigali Amendment to the Montreal Protocol (see Chapter 1). Due to environmental concerns, some countries have promoted switching from pMDIs to DPIs and slow mist inhalers (SMIs) as part of a sustainable strategy (26).

DISADVANTAGES OF A DPI

For Patients

Some patients with asthma and COPD are unable to completely disaggregate the powder within the DPI due to an inability to inspire forcefully. This can be assessed by a suboptimal PIFr. Characteristics of patients with a suboptimal PIFr include older age, female sex, short stature, and Black race (10, 27, 28); these four patient characteristics are variables that also predict lower lung function. In addition, a reduced inspiratory capacity as percent predicted, a marker of lung hyperinflation that adversely affects inspiratory muscle strength, and maximal inspiratory pressure are additional predictors of suboptimal PIFr (10, 29).

How common is a suboptimal PIFr? Haughney et al. (27) reported that 6.3% of 994 adults with asthma had a PIFr < 30 liters/min against a high-resistance DPI. For stable outpatients with COPD, the reported prevalence of a PIFr < 60 liters/minute for low-to-medium high-resistance DPIs ranges from 19% to 84% (14). For a high-resistance DPI, Al-Showair et al. (30) reported a 57% prevalence of a PIFr < 30 liters/minute measured directly through the HandiHaler® (Boehringer Ingelheim Pharma GmbH & Co; Ingelheim, Germany) in 163 outpatients with COPD. In patients hospitalized for a COPD exacerbation with PIFr measured prior to discharge, the reported prevalence of a suboptimal PIFr is 32% to 68% for a medium-low resistance DPI and 21% for a high-resistance DPI (14, 31, 32). The wide prevalence ranges for suboptimal PIFr likely reflect differences in patient populations as well as timing and methods of measuring PIFr.

As most dry powder formulations are attached to a lactose carrier, some HCPs advise patients with lactose intolerance not to use lactose-containing DPIs to minimize the risk of a hypersensitivity reaction (33). User life is the time interval from the removal of the inhaler from its packing until the manufacturer can no longer assure drug stability (> 80% of the respirable drug must be available at the end of the user life). For DPIs, user life ranges from four months (formoterol/budesonide Easyhaler®) to three years (formoterol/budesonide Turbohaler®) (34). User-life information is provided in the "Instructions for Use" in the United States and "Patient Information Leaflet" in Europe.

For HCPs

Some HCPs may not appreciate that patients should inhale "hard and fast" when using a DPI. Ideally, HCPs will query the patient about the expected symptomatic benefit (i.e., Are you able to breathe easier?) with a dry powder bronchodilator. If the patient reports little or no improvement, it is important for the HCP to ask the patient to describe and/or demonstrate the inhalation technique. If possible, the HCP should measure PIF against the simulated resistance of a particular DPI to assess whether the patient is likely or unlikely to benefit (14).

PATIENT ERRORS USING A DPI

Numerous investigators as well as systematic reviews have described technique errors in DPI use in patients with asthma and COPD. In 2008, Lavorini et al. (35) identified 27 articles on the incorrect use of DPIs in the management of adult patients with asthma or COPD. The most frequent error—"No exhalation before inhalation"—was consistently observed with eight different DPIs. The second most frequent error—"No breath hold"—was observed with five of seven different DPIs (35). Certainly, errors were expected given the observation by the authors that as many as 25% of patients in these studies never received verbal instructions on the DPI technique (35).

In 2016, Sanchis et al. (36) analyzed inhaler errors in 130 groups of patients who were involved in 21,497 tests with DPIs between 1975 and 2014. Of these, 44% [confidence interval (CI), 34–54%] had acceptable inhalation technique, while 23% (CI, 18–29%) had poor technique (36). Analyses also included 52 study groups in which full information on error frequencies for all five essential steps for DPIs was available (Table 6.3). Failure to "breathe out completely" was the

Table 6.3: Frequencies of Errors for Five Essential Steps for DPI Use Involving Adults with Either Asthma or COPD[a]

Step	Action	Error Percentage
1	Prepare the device: uncap, load the device	25
2	Turn away from the inhaler and breathe out completely	45
3	Place teeth and lips around the mouthpiece to form a seal	8
4	Breathe in with a single brisk, deep inhalation	16
5	Hold the breath for 5 to 10 seconds or as long as possible	35

[a] Results based on 52 study groups of patients (36).

most common error that occurred in an average of 45% (CI, 40–51%) of patients (36). The next most frequent error was "failure to breath-hold" in 35% (CI, 31–39%) of individuals (36). If a DPI is shaken, tilted, or dropped after the dose is loaded, delivery can be reduced (37).

Although general information on errors with DPIs is important, data on specific DPIs are clinically useful. In 2017, Price et al. (38) reported that "Insufficient inspiratory effort" was the most common critical error in 3,660 patients with asthma, which was associated with "uncontrolled asthma" in those using the Turbuhaler® (adjusted odds ratio = 1.30) and Diskus® (adjusted odds ratio = 1.56) devices, along with an increased exacerbation rate. In addition, Jang et al. (39) reported critical handling errors with four different DPIs (41% for the Breezhaler®, 12.5% for the Diskus®, 27.8% for the Ellipta®, and 44.4% for the Genuair®) in a prospective study of 261 Korean patients with COPD.

CONCLUSIONS

All three types of DPIs—single-unit, multi-unit, and reservoir—are used throughout the world for the treatment of patients with asthma and COPD. Dry powder medications are available as both reliever/rescue and maintenance therapies. The patient should inhale forcefully, or "hard and fast," to create turbulent energy within the DPI to disaggregate (i.e., pull off) the medication from the lactose carrier and then break the powder formulation into small, respirable particles. The turbulent energy generated by the patient is determined by the patient's PIFr and the internal resistance of the specific DPI. Generally, optimal values for PIFr are ≥ 60 liters/minute for low-to-medium high-resistance DPIs and ≥ 30 liters/minute for high-resistance devices.

A major advantage of DPIs is breath actuation as no hand-breath coordination is required, as with pMDIs and SMIs. In addition, two or more different medications and/or combinations are available in many of the same DPIs, providing device familiarity and continuity for patients and HCPs. As some patients with asthma and COPD have a suboptimal PIFr, they may be unable to completely disaggregate the powder within the device. This can result in a reduced dose delivered into the lower respiratory tract and affect efficacy. Common patient errors using a DPI are failure to breathe out completely before inhaling and failure to breath-hold after complete inhalation.

REFERENCES

1. Stein SW, Thiel CG. The history of therapeutic aerosols: A chronological review. J Aerosol Med Pulm Drug Deliv 2017;30:20–41.
2. The Montreal Protocol on substances that deplete the ozone layer. [cited 2022 Apr 27]. Available from: https://www.state.gov/key-topics-office-of-environmental-quality-and-transboundary-issues/the-montreal-protocol-on-substances-that-deplete-the-ozone-layer/
3. Laube BL, Janssens HM, de Jongh FHC, et al. What the pulmonary specialist should know about the new inhalational therapies. Eur Respir J 2011;37:1308–1331.
4. Maggi L, Bruni R, Conte U. Influence of the moisture on the performance of a new dry powder inhaler. Int J Pharm 1999;177:83–91.

5. USP 32. General notices and requirements: Applying to standards, tests, assays, and other specifications of the United States Pharmacopeia. [cited 2022 Mar 7]. Available from: https://www.usp.org/sites/default/files/usp_pd/EN/USPNF/generalNoticesandRequirementsFinal.pdf

6. Everard ML, Devadason SG, LeSouef PN. Flow early in the inspiratory manoever affects the aerosol particle size distribution from a Turbuhaler. Respir Med 1997;91:624–628.

7. Sanders MJ. Guiding inspiratory flow development of the In-Check DIAL G16, a tool for improving Inhaler technique. Pulm Med 2017;2017:1495867.

8. Yokoyama H, Yamamura Y, Ozeki T, et al. Analysis of relationship between peak inspiratory flow rate and amount of drug delivered to lungs following inhalation of fluticasone propionate with a Diskhaler. Biol Pharm Bull 2007;30:162–164.

9. Abdelrahim ME, Assi KH, Chrystyn H. Dose emission and aerodynamic characterization of the terbutaline sulfate dose emitted from a Turbuhaler at low inhalation flow. Pharm Dev Technol 2013;18:944–949.

10. Mahler DA. The role of inspiratory flow in selection and use of inhaled therapy for patients with chronic obstructive pulmonary disease. Respir Med 2020;161:105857.

11. Cooper A, Parker J, Berry M, et al. Wixela Inhub: Dosing performance *in vitro* and inhaled flow rates in healthy subjects and patients compared with Advair Diskus. J Aerosol Med Pulm Drug Deliv 2020;33:323–341.

12. Haidl P, Heindl S, Siemon K, et al. Inhalation device requirements for patients' inhalational maneuvers. Respir Med 2016;118:65–75.

13. Ghosh S, Ohar JA, Drummond MB. Peak inspiratory flow rate in chronic obstructive pulmonary disease: Implications for dry powder inhalers. J Aerosol Med Pulm Drug Deliv 2017;30:381–387.

14. Mahler DA, Halpin DMG. Peak inspiratory flow as a predictive therapeutic biomarker in COPD. Chest 2021;160:491–498.

15. Mahler DA. Peak inspiratory flow rate as a criterion for dry powder inhaler use in chronic obstructive pulmonary disease. Ann Am Thorac Soc 2017;14:1103–1107.

16. Magnussen H, Watz H, Zimmermann I, et al. Peak inspiratory flow through the Genuair® Inhaler in patients with moderate or severe COPD. Respir Med 2009;103:1832–1837.

17. Mahler DA. COPD: Answers to your most pressing questions about chronic obstructive pulmonary disease. Baltimore (MD): Johns Hopkins University Press; 2022. p. 78.

18. Chrystyn H, Niederlaender C. The Genuair® inhaler: A novel, multidose dry powder. Int J Clin Pract 2012;3:309–317.

19. Corradi M, Chrystyn H, Cosio BG, et al. NEXThaler, an innovative dry powder inhaler delivering an extrafine fixed combination of beclomethasone and formoterol to treat large and small airways in asthma. Expert Opin Drug Deliv 2014;11:1497–1506.

20. Reddel HK, FitzGerald JM, Bateman ED, et al. GINA 2019: A fundamental change in asthma management: Treatment of asthma with short-acting bronchodilators alone is no longer recommended for adults and adolescents. Eur Respir J 2019;53:1901046.

21. Reddel HK, Bacharier LB, Bateman ED, et al. Global initiative for asthma strategy 2021: Executive summary and rationale for key changes. Am J Respir Crit Care Med 2022;205:17–35.

22. Global Initiative for Chronic Obstructive Lung Disease. Global strategy for the diagnosis, management, and prevention of chronic obstructive pulmonary disease. 2022 report. [cited 2022 Sept 21]. Available from: https://goldcopd.org/2022-gold-reports-2

23. Nici L, Mammen MJ, Charbek E, et al. Pharmacologic management of chronic obstructive pulmonary disease. An official American Thoracic Society clinical practice guideline. Am J Respir Crit Care Med 2020;201:e56–e69.

24. Bourbeau J, Bhutani MN, Hernandez P, et al. Canadian Thoracic Society clinical practice guideline on pharmacotherapy in patients with COPD – 2019 update of evidence. Can J Respir Crit Care Sleep Med 2019;3(9):1–23. DOI:10.1080/24745332.2019.1668652

25. Miravitlles M, Calle M, Molina J, et al. Spanish COPD guidelines (GesEPOC) 2021: Updated pharmacological treatment of stable COPD. Arch Bronchoneumol 2022;58:69–81.

26. British Thoracic Society. Environment and lung health position statement, 2020. [updated 2022 10 Feb; cited 2022 Mar 7]. Available from: https://www.brit-thoracic.org.uk/aboutus/goverance-documents-and-policies/position-statements/

27. Haughney J, Lee AJ, McKnight E, et al. Peak inspiratory flow measured at different inhaler resistances in patients with asthma. J Allergy Clin Immunol Pract 2021;9:890–896.

28. Mahler DA, Niu X, Deering KL, et al. Prospective evaluation of exacerbations associated with suboptimal peak inspiratory flow among stable outpatients with COPD. Int J Chron Obstruct Pulmon Dis 2022;17:559–568.

29. Van der Palen J. Peak inspiratory flow through Diskus and Turbuhaler, measured by means of a peak inspiratory flow meter (In-Chck DIAL®). Respir Med 2003;97:285–289.

30. Al-Showair RAM, Tarsin WY, Assi KH, et al. Can all patients with COPD use the correct inhalation flow with all inhalers and does training help? Respir Med 2007;101:2395–2401.

31. Clark B, Wells BJ, Saha AK, et al. Low peak inspiratory flow rates are common among COPD inpatients and are associated with increased healthcare resource utilization: A retrospective cohort study. Int J Chron Obstruct Pulmon Dis 2022;17:1483–1494.

32. Mahler DA, Demirel S, Hollander R, et al. High prevalence of suboptimal peak inspiratory flow in hospitalized patients with COPD: A real-world study. Chronic Obstr Pulm Dis 2022;17:559–568.

33. Robles J, Motheral L. Hypersensitivity reaction after inhalation of a lactose-containing dry powder inhaler. J Pediatr Pharmacol Ther 2014;19:206–211.

34. Pleasants RA, Tilley SL, Hickey AJ, et al. User-life of ICS/LABA inhaler devices should be considered when prescribed as relievers. Eur Respir J 2021;57:2003921.

35. Lavorini F, Magnan A, Dubus JC, et al. Effect of incorrect use of dry powder inhalers on management of patients with asthma and COPD. Respir Med 2008;102:593–604.

36. Sanchis J, Gich I, Pedersen S. Systematic review of errors in inhaler use: Has patient technique improved over time? Chest 2016;150:394–406.

37. Kondo T, Tanigaki T, Yokoyama H, et al. Impact of holding position during inhalation on drug release from a reservoir-, blister-, and capsule-type dry powder inhaler. J Asthma 2017;54:792–737.
38. Price DB, Roman-Rodriguez M, McQueen RB, et al. Inhaler errors in the CRITIKAL study: Type, frequency, and association with asthma outcomes. J Allergy Clin Immunol Pract 2017;5:1071–1081.
39. Jang JG, Chung JH, Shin KC, et al. Comparative study of inhaler device handling technique and risk factors for critical inhaler errors in Korean COPD patients. Int J Chron Obstruct Pulmon Dis 2021;16:1051–1059.

7 Digital Inhalers for the Management of Obstructive Lung Diseases

Roy A. Pleasants and Stephen L. Tilley

CONTENTS

INTRODUCTION

Nonadherence and improper inhaler technique are major contributors to poor outcomes in patients with asthma and chronic obstructive pulmonary disease (COPD) (1–4). Reasons for such behaviors are multifactorial, including self-treatment of a variable, symptom-based disease. It is well documented that physician assessment is little better than chance (3, 4) at judging patient's adherence with inhalers, and self- and parental reports often overestimate treatments actually taken (5). Inhaler technique is frequently suboptimal and even when properly taught, patients need retraining (2, 6).

To address these problems, inhalers have been reengineered with digital sensors to detect proper use by patients (7). Attachable or embedded electromechanical sensors record and wirelessly transmit data showing when and how patients use their inhalers. When applied to patient care, they are termed digital inhaler health solutions. These devices came to the market about 10 years ago to improve medication adherence (8). Most clinical studies report that using digital inhalers improves care in COPD and asthma patients, adolescents, and older patients. With the rapid expansion of telehealth in the outpatient setting, ongoing gaps in inhaler use, costs associated with uncontrolled obstructive lung diseases, and organizations and payers increasingly supportive of digital telehealth, it is projected the global digital inhaler market will be in the billions of US dollars before 2030 (9).

In this chapter, we present an overview of the different components and applications of the digital inhaler health solution. This includes the devices, platform components, clinical evidence, privacy and security issues, and finally the patient and physician interfaces in applying this to care.

DIGITAL INHALER PLATFORM

Figure 7.1 shows a digital platform consisting of inhaler(s) with sensors, the patient, smartphone and dedicated app, the healthcare professional (HCP), and their dashboard portal (8). Remote patient monitoring (RPM) occurs

DOI: 10.1201/9781003269014-7

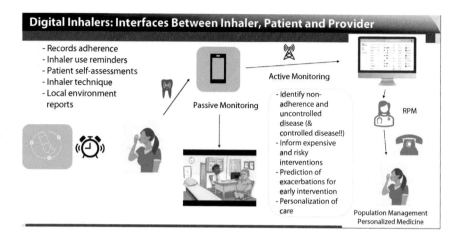

Figure 7.1 Digital Inhaler Health Platform. RPM = remote patient monitoring.

when the HCP accesses digital data through their dashboard portal to help guide care. When the HCP has real-time access to the patient's inhaler use, it is termed active RPM. With passive RPM, the same data are still recorded and ultimately available. Alternating between active and passive monitoring of inhaler use might be employed. Depending on the specific digital inhaler product, the clinician can review the patient's adherence, assess the inhaler technique, evaluate recorded patient-reported outcomes (PRO), and generate reports for review and documentation. Integration into the electronic health record will ultimately connect inhaler data with other aspects of care more readily.

Description of Devices

Table 7.1 describes common, available digital inhalers. Electronic sensors are either attached (CapMedic®, Hallie®, INCA, Propeller Health, Amiko Respiro®) or embedded in the inhaler (Respiro RSX01, Teva Digihaler®). With each inhaler actuation, an electronic sensor time stamps and records use, stores these data for a finite time, and transmits the data when a paired mobile device is in close proximity. Sensors rely on pressure changes, audio, or vibration for such measurements (8, 10). A radar sensor transmits data via Bluetooth® technology. While devices can record each actuation, they do not ensure the patient receives a therapeutic dose, such as when pressing the attached sensor without inhaling, or if the product is compromised, such as past-expiry.

To help guide inhaler technique, inspiratory-capable (IC) sensors for pressurized metered dose inhaler (pMDI) and dry powder inhalers (DPI) can measure flows (Capmedic®, Digihaler®, Adherium Hailie® for Symbicort® pMDI, and Amiko Respiro®) and others detect proper shaking or upright position for pMDIs (Capmedic®, Hailie®). With Digihaler®, the patient can see whether they achieved the proper inspiration categorically, while with CapMedic®, flashing lights and audio coach the patient. The patient and clinician may consider this feedback on technique as a value-added function, rather than solely monitoring adherence. Notably, sensors that detect shaking are available for pMDIs (Hailie®, Capmedic®), but no sensor warns about shaking DPIs, known to decrease dose delivery (11).

Table 7.1: Currently Available Digital Inhaler Devices

Digital Inhaler Name Manufacturer	Description Sensors	Inhaler Compatibility	Clinician Interface	Patient Interface	Photos of Devices and Inhalers
Capmedic® Cognita Labs, LLC Houston, TX	Records each actuation Companion digital device to measure PEF and FEV1	Most pMDIs in US including Ventolin®, Proair®, Symbicort®, Advair® Flovent®, Dulera®, Atrovent®)	Portal dashboard reporting patient's inhaler use and lung function when measured by a companion spirometer (FEV1, PEF)	Track medication use and inhaler technique on app Vocally coaches for correct inhaler use based on inhaler shaking, orientation, coordination, duration of inhalation, and breath-hold	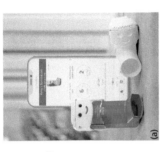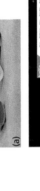 (a)
Hailie® Adherium LLC, Auckland, NZ	Records each actuation Attachable sensors Depending on device, detects actuation by pressure, temperature, acoustics	Compatible with most pMDIs and DPIs including Diskus®, Turbuhaler®, Handihaler®, Symbicort® pMDI, Ventolin®, Proair®, Dulera®, Atrovent® pMDI), Bevespi® MDI	Portal dashboard reporting patient's inhaler use and lung function when measured by a companion spirometer (PEF)	Smartphone dashboard Audible, scheduled alerts from sensor Patient can input PEF if measured by companion device	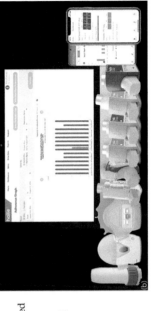 (b)

(Continued)

Table 7.1: Currently Available Digital Inhaler Devices (Continued)

Digital Inhaler Name Manufacturer	Description Sensors	Inhaler Compatibility	Clinician Interface	Patient Interface	Photos of Devices and Inhalers
Respiro® Amiko Milan, Italy	Records each actuation and inhalational flow for DPI and pMDI Attachable, electromechanical sensors Built-in sensors for RSX01	Compatible with most pMDIs and DPIs including Accuhaler®, Turbuhaler®, Handihaler®	Portal dashboard reporting patient's inhaler use and inhalational flows Reports with trends of inhaler use and clinical data entered by a patient	Smartphone dashboard Audible, scheduled alerts from the sensor and/or smartphone	(c) (d)

(Continued)

Table 7.1: Currently Available Digital Inhaler Devices (Continued)

Digital Inhaler Name Manufacturer	Description Sensors	Inhaler Compatibility	Clinician Interface	Patient Interface	Photos of Devices and Inhalers
Propeller sensors Propeller Health, Madison WI, Respironics	Attachable, electromechanical sensors	Compatible with most pMDIs (e.g., Ventolin®, Symbicort® pMDI); SMIs (Respimat®), and DPIs (Diskus®, Turbuhaler®, Handihaler®, Ellipta®)	Portal dashboard reporting patient's inhaler use Reports trends of inhaler use and clinical data entered by a patient Environmental daily reports	Smartphone dashboard Audible, scheduled alerts from the attached sensor Alerts on worsening Environmental reports	(e)
Digihaler® Teva Pharm Tel Aviv, Israel	Records each actuation and inhalational flow Embedded sensors measuring pressure changes in airflow	US ProAir Digihaler® (albuterol) Armonair Digihaler® (Fluticasone) Airduo Digihaler® (Fluticasone/ Salmeterol) Europe Symbicort Digihaler® (Under development)	Portal dashboard reporting patient's inhaler use and inhalational flows (aids inhaler technique and provides a physiologic measure) Reports with trends of inhaler use and clinical data entered by a patient	Smartphone dashboard Audible, scheduled alerts from sensor App alerts on worsening, refills Local environmental reports	(f)

Abbreviations: DPI = dry powder inhaler; FEV1 = forced expiratory volume in 1 second; PEF = peak expiratory flow; pMDI = pressurized metered dose inhaler; SMI = soft mist inhaler.

(Continued)

Regulatory Approval

The US Food and Drug Administration (FDA) and European Medicines Agency (EMA) provide guidance to manufacturers of attachable devices and inhalers with embedded sensors (12–15). In Europe, software specifically developed for the diagnosis or treatment of disease falls under the medical device directive. The FDA provides specific guidance on premarket submissions of software combined/contained in medical devices. Prior to marketing, attachable digital inhaler sensors must meet regulatory standards for devices (510K in the US), and if built directly into the inhaler, both drug and device regulations apply (combination product). In addition to device approval, associated software must go through regulatory review and approval (16). In the US, the Digital Health Center of Excellence, part of the Center for Devices and Radiological Health, serves as a resource for regulatory advice and support to the FDA (17). The FDA also regulates medical apps, defined as apps intended to be used as "accessory to a regulated medical device" or having the ability to "transform a mobile platform into a regulated medical device." Apps that do not satisfy this definition are designated health apps and are not regulated as such.

Attachable sensors do not have to demonstrate clinical efficacy; rather, device safety is the priority, including not interfering with inhaler operation, medication delivery, or obstructing the dose counter or label. Both the built-in and attachable electronic monitoring devices for digital inhalers are considered low risk (Class II, US FDA). The Digihaler®, a combination product, was approved as a New Drug Application and device through the Center for Devices and Radiologic Health (18). For Digihaler®, several other federal agencies were involved in the review process for the app including cybersecurity and patient-facing materials.

PRIVACY AND CYBERSECURITY

Privacy and security are a concern for patients and HCPs due to sharing of sensitive personal and health data on smartphones and the internet (19–21). The American College of Physicians advocates that protected health information be secure from improper access or use, and supports an environment of trust while improving care (22). Factors affecting an individual's willingness to share personal health data include the user's motive, perceived benefits, and the sensitivity of the information (20). Healthcare systems considering digital inhalers will want to address any cybersecurity issues and likely require an in-depth review prior to implementation. Remote digital device monitoring in cardiac diseases and diabetes may serve as models.

Digital inhaler device manufacturers must adhere to privacy standards set forth by regulators such as the US FDA and EMA. Cybersecurity with medical devices undergoes rigorous regulatory assessment, and multiple agencies are involved. US Federal regulations, called quality system regulations, require that medical device manufacturers address risks during development and post-marketing (17). In the US, all transfer of data is encrypted and secured according to standards set by the National Institute of Standards and Technology and Security Operations Center.

User Agreements on the mobile app inform patients about data aggregation and de-identification and may include sharing for public health and scientific research. The Privacy Policy explains how personal and health information is collected, stored, disclosed, and transferred when any element of digital services is used. These must meet the Health Insurance, Portability, and Accountability Act (HIPAA) regulations, whether by a covered entity (HCP) or non-covered entity (20). The minimum data required are name, smartphone number, mailing address, and email address in order to e-consent. Additional health (e.g., HCP info) and personal information (medications, triggers) is required to use all platform elements. Parental or guardian consent is required for minors.

Patient and Provider Interfaces

After enrolling in the digital inhaler platform, patients can use their mobile app to review inhaler use over time and receive inhaler technique feedback if available. Depending on the capabilities of the app, additional interface occurs, such as patients to record patient-reported outcomes (PROs) or reviewing local environment reports. All devices provide audible and/or visual alerts to remind patients to use their maintenance inhalers; this function can be activated and deactivated. Patients may also receive messages such as the need to resync and alerts to contact their HCP with excess short-acting β-2 agonist (SABA) use. Digital inhalers that assist with inhaler technique provide feedback on the smartphone dashboard, and sometimes visually or from sensors. In terms of usability and perceived value, digital inhalers have been well received by asthmatics and COPD patients enrolled in clinical studies (20, 23–25).

HCP can use the dashboard portal to review enrollee's data to monitor inhaler use for clinical care, assess the need for follow-up (depending on the predefined digital inhaler strategy), and generate reports for documentation and billing. The frequency of review and the HCP's response are based on the clinical plan discussed with the patient.

Attrition occurs with digital inhaler use, by as much as 40% of patients in the first 6 months (26) and 55% in 1 year (27). Reasons include device malfunction, loss of interest, concerns about intrusiveness, and perhaps because patients do not want to share their growing non-adherence. One study in adults found a small percentage (5.3%) of devices malfunctioned with use (28), while pediatric studies reported higher rates of snap-on device loss or damage (29, 30).

CLINICAL EVIDENCE

Studies in asthma and COPD support the use of digital inhalers in the outpatient setting among adults and children to improve adherence and clinical outcomes (24, 27, 29, 31–35). Importantly, these studies provide a greater understanding of patient behaviors using inhalers and more objective evidence of the role of adherence on patient outcomes. Table 7.2 describes peer-reviewed, randomized, prospective studies of digital inhalers, assessing the impact on outcomes, adherence with controllers and relievers, need for acute care visits, and PROs. Table 7.3 shows studies evaluating the use of digital inhalers to predict exacerbations.

Identifying Rescue and Maintenance Inhaler Patterns

Digital inhaler studies have better-characterized inhaler usage patterns with relievers and controllers (36, 37) than shown with databases or patient self-report. Assessment of SABA use is recommended in current guidelines as a measure of disease control for asthma and COPD (38–40), as overuse of SABA is related to increased morbidity and mortality (5, 41). In a prospective study of 58 COPD patients using digital inhalers, four SABA use patterns were found: 1) frequent use, regular pattern, 2) frequent use, no pattern, 3) infrequent users, and 4) infrequent, but intense use (36). Groups 2 and 3 were the most common use patterns and rescue inhaler use compelled by symptoms. Frequent inhaler use with no pattern was associated with more symptoms compared with frequent use with a regular daily pattern. A prospective study in 32 COPD

Table 7.2: Studies of Digital Inhalers Reporting Clinical Outcomes

Study Design Duration	Setting Study Population Study Group(s)	Digital Device Drug(s)	Patient and Clinician Interface with EMD and Apps	Primary Outcome	Secondary Outcome
Chan (2015) RCT 6 months	Pediatric Specialty Children with asthma aged 6–15 yr on ICS (n=220) with recent exacerbation requiring ED EMD+BF vs Usual care	Adherium SmartTrack® ICS pMDI Albuterol pMDI	Patient adherence reminders by device	Medication adherence: 84% with EMD vs 30% in the control group (p<0.0001) No difference in school absenteeism	↑asthma score with EMD Improvement in comorbidity score (p=0.008) Child ACT (p<0.001) improved in EMD+BF Lower SABA use in EMD+BF(p=0.002) No effect on FEV1
Mosnaim (2020) R, single-blinded	Allergy clinic Adults with uncontrolled asthma (n=100) EMD + BF vs Usual care with passive EMD 14 weeks	Propeller Health ICS and SABA pMDI	Yes	↑ in SABA-free days = 19% for EMD+ BF vs 6% in the control group (passive EMD)	ICS adherence over 14 weeks = −2% EMD+BF vs −17% in control group
Merchant (2016) RCT, parallel arms	Allergy clinic Children and adults with asthma > 5 years old (n=495) EMD + BF vs Usual care 12 months	Propeller Health Albuterol pMDI	Clinician access to dashboard Personalized feedback to the patient via mobile phone app	↑SABA free days in EMD+BF vs usual care group +17% vs +21%, p<0.01	↑ in ACT with EMD+BF vs control group (+6.2 vs +4.6 p<0.01)

(Continued)

Table 7.2: Studies of Digital Inhalers Reporting Clinical Outcomes (Continued)

Study Design Duration	Setting Study Population Study Group(s)	Digital Device Drug(s)	Patient and Clinician Interface with EMD and Apps	Primary Outcome	Secondary Outcome
Foster (2014) RCT 6 months	Primary Care Adults with mod / severe asthma based on ACT (n=143) EMD + BF vs Adherence discussion only vs Usual care 6 months	Adherium Smarttrack® ICS/LABA (Accuhaler®) Albuterol pMDI	Patient Inhaler reminders with Clinician dashboard prompting patient contact with suboptimal inhaler adherence	No difference in ACT among three groups	Adherence in EMD+BF = 74%, usual care = 46%; discussion only group = 46% ↓ exacerbation rates with inhaler reminders (11% vs 28%) No difference in other PRO or FEV1 among three groups
O'Dwyer (2016) RCT, parallel	Pharmacies were unit of randomization Community pharmacists assisted with digital inhalers	INCA® ICS/LABA Accuhaler®	EMD + BF	↑Adherence 60.8% in EMD + BF + Inhaler instruction vs 44.2% in Inhaler instruction only vs 33.2% in usual care	SGRQ (−6.1) in EMD + BF group at 2 and 6 months Inhaler training group had improvement at 2 months, but not at 6 months
Morton (2017) RCT, Open-label	Pediatric asthma 6–16 years old (n=77) Intervention group (EMD with controller reminders and review of adherence at clinic visits 1 year	Adherium Smartinhaler(R), Smartturbo(R) ICS pMDI and ICS DPI SABA pMDI	Passive recording of EMD use Adherence reviewed at clinic visits with HCP	No difference in ACQ(p=0.35)	Adherence improved in intervention group 70% vs 49% (p=0.001) ↓ exacerbations in intervention (p=0.008) and hospitalizations (p<0.001) No difference in SABA use, FEV1, or PAQLQ or asthma severity

(Continued)

Table 7.2: Studies of Digital Inhalers Reporting Clinical Outcomes (Continued)

Study Design Duration	Setting Study Population Study Group(s)	Digital Device Drug(s)	Patient and Clinician Interface with EMD and Apps	Primary Outcome	Secondary Outcome
Sulaiman (2018) RCT	Pulmonary Clinic Adults with severe asthma and exacerbations in last year (n=360) Control (Intensive education = technique and adherence) vs Intervention (Intensive education + BF from EMD) 3 months	INCA (Seretide®)	BF via monthly nurse visits in Intervention Group	73% of adherence (frequency of use, correct technique) in EMD+BF vs 63% in control group (p<0.01)	PEF at 3 months NSS between groups ACT or AQLQ NSS between groups
Gregoriano (2019) Single-blind RCT	Pulmonary clinic Adult asthma and COPD with exacerbation in the last year (n=149) 6 months	Smartinhaler® Albuterol pMDI Controllers DPI	EMD with Clinician dashboard + BF. (Patient inhaler alerts, Clinician assessments) vs Passive EMD	No effect on time to first exacerbation (HR 0.65, 95% CI 0.21–2.07, p=0.024)	Trend in decreased exacerbation frequency (RR=0.61, CI=0.35–1.03, p=0.07) Days adherent > in intervention group (pMDI 82±14% vs 60±30%, p,0.01) And DPI controllers (90±10% vs 80±21%, p=0.01) No effects on SGRQ
Jochmann 2021 Open-label, Proof of Concept study	Pediatric Pulmonary Clinic Pediatric Asthma (n=35) previously enrolled in passive digital inhaler study, 6 months	Smartinhaler® ICS	Patients enrolled in prior passive EMD study switched to either active monitoring or continued on passive EMD Dashboard not employed	No effect on adherence (78% vs 83%, p=0.304) Improvement in PROs with active intervention	Not specified Difficulties with 10 inhalers unable to download smartphone data. Seven subjects lost their digital sensor

(Continued)

Table 7.2: Studies of Digital Inhalers Reporting Clinical Outcomes (Continued)

Study Design Duration	Setting Study Population Study Group(s)	Digital Device Drug(s)	Patient and Clinician Interface with EMD and Apps	Primary Outcome	Secondary Outcome
Criner 2021 Phase 4, Randomized, open-label trial	Eight research sites in US including pulmonary clinics Mod-severe COPD (*n*=138) 6 months	Smartinhaler® ICS/LABA	Patients randomized to passive EMD with daily sensors reminders vs passive EMD with no reminders Dashboard not employed	Adherence improved with reminders (77.6% vs 60.2%; *p*<0.001)	None reported 17% of devices not connected at 28 days, because devices were uploaded and synced by patients without direct supervision
Moore 2021 Open-label, parallel-group RCT	Multi-national clinic study Uncontrolled adult asthma (*n*=437) 6 months	ICS/LABA SABA	Randomized to five groups based on data feedback from device and/or prescriber Dashboard applied in active feedback by prescriber group	Mean(SD) adherence 82.2% (16.8) in the maintenance to participants and HCPs arm vs 70.8(27.3)% in the control Difference of 12.0% SS(95% CI: 5.2–18.8%; *p*,0.001) Adherence also significantly greater in other arms vs Control	Mean SABA-free days (months 4–6) significantly greater in those who received data on rescue use vs control ACT scores improved in all study arms – NSS between groups

Abbreviations: ACQ = Asthma Control Questionnaire; Asthma ACT = Asthma Control Test; AQLQ = Asthma Quality of Life Questionnaire; BF = biofeedback; COPD = chronic obstructive pulmonary disease; DPI = dry powder inhaler; EMD = electronic monitoring device; FEV1 = forced expiratory volume in 1 second; HCP = healthcare professional; ICS = inhaled corticosteroid; LABA = long-acting β-2 agonist; NSS = not statistically significant; PEF = peak expiratory flow; pMDI = pressurized metered dose inhaler; PAQLQ = Pediatric Asthma Quality of Life Questionnaire; PRO = patient-reported outcome; RCT = randomized clinical trial; SABA = short-acting β-2 agonist; SD = standard deviation; SGRQ = St George Respiratory Questionnaire; SMI = slow mist inhaler.

Table 7.3: Use of Digital Inhalers to Predict Acute Events in Asthma and COPD Patients

Author (Year) Design	Study Population Study Group(s) Duration	Digital Device Drug(s)	Outcome Measures	Outcome
Killane (2016) RCT, parallel group	Adults with asthma (n = 184) EMD + Inhaler teaching vs Inhaler teaching only 3 months	INCA ICS/LABA – Accuhaler® Clinician assessment of medication adherence by EMD recordings at monthly study visits Clinician feedback to subject at study visits regarding adherence	Exacerbation risk	< 80% adherence by EMD predictive of AECOPD
Pleasants (2019) Prospective open-label	Adults with asthma (n = 360) on ICS/LABA with exacerbation in prior year Passive EMD 24 weeks	Teva Digihaler® Albuterol	Clinical, β-2 agonist use, and inspiratory flow measures to predict exacerbations using machine learning modeling	PIF and inhalation volume measured by Digihaler decline with exacerbations Albuterol use increases with exacerbations.
Snyder (2020) Prospective open-label	COPD with a history of exacerbation (n = 336) 24 weeks	Teva Digihaler® Albuterol DPI	Clinical, B-agonist use, and inspiratory flow measures to predict exacerbations	PIF and inhalation volume measured by Digihaler decline with exacerbations Albuterol use increases with exacerbations
Sumino (2018) Prospective observational	COPD (n = 35) 12 weeks	Propeller Albuterol pMDI Passive EMD without dashboard	Exacerbation risk based on albuterol use compared to baseline	Odds ratio of an exacerbation 1.54 (1.21–1.97 with ↑ albuterol use > 100%
Patel (2013) RCT, secondary analysis using nested cohort	Severe asthma (n = 303) 24 weeks	Adherium Albuterol pMDI and ICS/FOR DPI Passive EMD without dashboard	Albuterol use to predict exacerbations	Each associated with an increased risk of future severe exacerbation Higher mean daily albuterol use (OR 1.24) Higher days of albuterol use (OR 1.15) Higher maximal 24-h use (OR 1.09)

patients found that the majority (73%) of SABA over-users were on guideline-concordant therapies, while 27% of the over-users were not (37).

SABA use is known to increase around exacerbations, but now we have more objective evidence. One digital inhaler study reported that increased SABA use from baseline (100%), rather than the number of puffs, was most predictive of an ensuing exacerbation in asthma and COPD (25). In a study employing albuterol Digihaler®, increased SABA use was observed about 5 days prior to receipt of systemic corticosteroids in adult asthmatics (mean 2.2–4.0 puffs/day), then declined to baseline over a similar timeframe (42). In a similar study on COPD, albuterol use changed around exacerbations to a lesser extent (mean 3.3–4.3 puffs/day) (43). A downside of digital inhalers is the inability to document nebulizer use; a third of COPD patients use nebulizers acutely or chronically (44).

Characterizing maintenance inhaler use may identify patients for whom interventions for non-adherence would improve outcomes; as well as patients who are controlled, but non-adherent. Studies using digital inhalers have objectively identified different patterns of maintenance adherence (30, 45–48). Employing a digital inhaler that records use and inhaler technique, four adherence patterns in COPD were identified: 1) regular use, good technique, 2) regular use, frequent critical inhaler error, 3) irregular use, good technique, and 4) irregular use, frequent critical errors (49). In a study of pediatric asthmatics monitored for a median of 92 days, the median (range) monitored adherence was 74% (21–99%). They identified four groups: 1) good adherence during monitoring with improved control, 24%; 2) good adherence with poor control, 18% (severe therapy-resistant asthma); 3) poor adherence with good control, 26%; and 4) poor adherence with poor control, 32% (30).

Controller Adherence in the Clinical Setting

Adherence to inhaled medications in asthma and COPD is the lowest among common chronic diseases, in part related to symptom variability and quick response to bronchodilators (3). Based on pharmacy claims data, regular use of daily maintenance medications is often <50% in patients with asthma (50) and COPD (51). Clinicians commonly overestimate adherence to inhaled therapies. In one study, digital records of adherence were more accurate than relying on a dose counter (52). Studies in asthma and COPD (4, 53, 54) support the regular use of maintenance inhalers (termed adherent and controlled), and this is the basis for clinicians to promote the daily use of controllers. On the other hand, the definition of optimal adherence continues to change in asthma, whereas the needed use of ICS or ICS/FOR is increasingly being shown to be as effective as regular use in some asthmatics (55).

Most studies demonstrate that digital inhaler use improves medication adherence, defined by decreased rescue inhaler use and regular use of controllers (27, 31–35, 56, 57). Compared to passive adherence monitoring, the effect is greater in patients with biofeedback through reminder alerts and active clinician monitoring (Table 7.2) (31–34, 56). A randomized control trial in 437 uncontrolled adult asthmatics evaluated the effect of direct biofeedback over 24 weeks on inhaler adherence. The study found that in the group with biofeedback using a smartphone app, adherence to DPI increased by 82%, compared to 69% in a control group with passive monitoring (31). Two studies reported improved adherence using the dashboard throughout the study to provide feedback (33, 58). Another study in 100 uncontrolled adult asthmatics found over a period of 14 weeks that ICS adherence declined less with the use of digital inhalers (2%) than in the control group (17%) who did not receive reminders or feedback on medication use (32). Other studies found more substantial improvements in controller adherence with digital inhalers (28, 33, 56–58), but baseline adherence was poor. These data indicate that patients already adherent with controllers are less likely to benefit from digital inhalers that simply document adherence.

Role in Exacerbations

In addition to reducing exacerbations by improving controller adherence and greater patient engagement, digital inhalers may help identify clinical worsening. In two prospective, observational studies with IC-albuterol Digihaler®, a post-hoc machine learning model using inhaler use frequency and inhalation measures was able to predict an ensuing exacerbation (receiver operating curve - asthma 0.79 and COPD 0.81) (42, 43). Albuterol use increased most evidently 5 days prior to the exacerbation; the same pattern was found in asthmatics using digitalized budesonide/formoterol DPI as needed (Maintenance and Reliever Therapy) (59).

A potential role of IC-digital inhalers could be the ability to provide ambulatory lung function measures, specifically peak inspiratory flow (PIF) and inhaled volume (Vin), analogous to peak expiratory flow monitoring. Studies using spirometry or a portable inspiratory device (InCheckDial®) show PIF (60, 61, 62) and Vin are bronchodilator responsive (62–64) and change with clinical worsening in asthma and COPD (59, 65, 66). Using the IC-albuterol Digihaler®, studies in asthma and COPD showed both the mean Vin and PIF decreased during outpatient exacerbations, the former to a greater extent (asthma 18% vs 12%, COPD 16% vs 9%, respectively) (42, 43). For the IC-Digihaler®, the recommended full expiration followed by a full inspiration yields a maximum inspiratory flow and Vin. For pMDIs, the recommended slow and forceful exhalation followed by a deep slow inhalation through the inhaler yields Vin. The sensors are accurate if used properly (67–69).

Inhaler Adherence in Clinical Drug Trials

Digital inhalers should be considered for use in drug trials to quantify inhaler use and lessen the impact of non-adherence on results (70, 71). In an analysis of 87 randomized clinical trials of add-on therapy in severe asthma, none had objective evidence of inhaler adherence (72). Patient self-report of adherence is prone to overestimation due to social desirability bias (5). Mechanical dose-counters on inhalers are often used to measure adherence in trials but overestimate actual use compared with adherence measurements by digital inhalers (52).

APPLYING DIGITAL INHALERS TO CLINICAL PRACTICE
Patient Selection

To employ digital inhalers, the HCP should first determine if there are any barriers such as cost or side effects that limit use of the medication to be digitalized. Importantly, the HCP should determine if RPM is reimbursable since not all US payers consider these codes billable. They should determine if and how the patient uses a nebulizer to understand how a digital inhaler fits into the patient's inhaled medications. Although not necessary, ideally the patient must possess and know how to operate a smartphone. Table 7.4 shows representative patient types that may benefit from a digital inhaler health solution. Benefits from using digital inhalers arise principally from improved adherence to maintenance inhalers, while monitoring rescue inhalers serves as a surrogate for uncontrolled disease. Optimizing the inhaler technique could help any of the proposed patient types but should be done in conjunction with adherence monitoring.

Table 7.4: Patients Who May Benefit from a Digital Inhaler Health Solution

Uncontrolled asthma or COPD in outpatient setting despite optimal prescriptions
Considering addition of costly interventions such as biologics or procedures
Considering risky interventions such as biopsy or costly radiology for alternative
 diagnosis
Post-acute care for exacerbation such as post-ED for asthma or post-hospital for COPD
Patient with suspected or known poor inhaler technique with suboptimal disease control
Use of ICS/FOR Maintenance and Reliever Therapy (MART) for asthma

Prescribing and Dispensing Devices

While not all inhaler sensors require a prescription, the HCP will initiate the process for patients to obtain the device. For attachable sensors, will agree contractually to purchase the devices including access to the cloud server. Attachable digital sensors can be dispensed at the clinician's site or sent by postal delivery to the patient. Digital inhalers with built-in sensors require a prescription; therefore, HCP should follow formulary procedures such as prior authorization and other dispensing requirements.

Informing and Enrolling the Patient

Digital inhalers will impact the patient, the HCP, and patient–HCP interactions. Typically, it will be the prescriber who will decide on the need for a digital inhaler, followed by a discussion with the patient. The intent of digital inhalers is to increase patient self-care and provide objective evidence of inhaler use, so the discussion should proceed on that basis. The patient should receive an overview of the devices and mobile app functions, how this may benefit their care, security and privacy issues, costs, goals, and the monitoring plan. Clinical responsibility for reviewing and acting on potentially continuous data streams needs to be very clear and documented on how the prescriber and patient will employ digital inhalers. A written action plan may be appropriate. Telling the patient to seek medical care as they normally would is a reasonable strategy, rather than relying on the prescriber to identify acute worsening prospectively. However, in the post-acute care period, desired monitoring may be daily. There is a paucity of data on whether such a model improves outcomes, only that inhaler use is suboptimal in this setting (47).

Enrolling a patient in a digital health solution is best done in-person or by video telehealth, where the provider can assist and instruct the patient. In one study of COPD patients, a significant number (17%) of technical failures occurred if patients attempted to complete enrollment on their own (35). The devices are easy to attach, it is the operation that may be complex. For prescription combination digital inhalers, a trained dispensing pharmacist could assist the patient with app download, device syncing, and operation.

After receiving the sensor, the patient downloads the manufacturer's companion app onto their smartphone, and they are required to e-consent to User and Privacy agreements. The agreements describe in detail how the data will be collected, transmitted, and utilized. The patient will not be able to use all platform functions without the use of a cloud server through their smartphone. An alternative for the patient without a smartphone or patients choosing not to share their data wirelessly is to bring their digital inhaler to in-person clinic visits and having the data uploaded. Some Adherium devices also have a USB port for download (Hailie Connect®).

PATIENT MONITORING

While the use of digital inhalers to provide reminder alerts and technique feedback has benefits, it must be acknowledged that changes in patient behavior may be limited for a variety of reasons. Rather, the greatest value of digital inhalers will be in understanding the patient's behavior and adapting treatments thereof.

The strategy and time interval for digital monitoring are part of the personalization of patient care. Based on current evidence, the time period needed to correctly assess maintenance inhaler adherence likely needs to be at least 3 months (73). The HCP's investment in time and resources should be considered. While one study of stable patients reported that 1 week of monitoring defined maintenance adherence (36), most studies followed patients for many months. In some studies, it was found that adherence improved, then declined over time, often becoming evident at about 3–6 months (31). Also not accounted for in these studies was seasonal variation in disease control.

Payers may influence the frequency of monitoring. In the US, the Committee on Medicare and Medicaid Services criteria for RPM permits billing as often as once monthly and must contain digitally collected data for 16 days/month. While feedback from the mobile app and digital inhaler is important for the patient to remain engaged, HCP feedback is necessary, and waiting too long will lead to dropouts.

CONCLUSIONS

Available for more than two decades, digital inhalers and associated health platforms remain new to many clinicians and healthcare organizations. A digital inhaler is described by whether it is an attachable device or a drug and device product combination, and whether it has the capability to guide inhaler technique by detecting inspiratory flow or shaking. When used as intended, digital inhaler data can be a powerful tool to engage patients in active discussions about their actual medication-taking behaviors, attitudes toward their prescribed treatments, and beliefs about their disease.

Most studies demonstrate that digital inhalers enhance medication management by improving adherence and clinical outcomes. Additional data are needed to show if devices improve inhaler technique and in whom and how long they should be employed. Digital inhalers represent a great opportunity to help solve some key problems with inhaler use.

ABBREVIATIONS

COPD	chronic obstructive pulmonary disease
DPI	dry powder inhaler
EMA	European Medicines Authority
FDA	Food and Drug Administration
HCP	healthcare professional
HIPAA	Health Insurance, Portability, and Accountability Act
IC	inspiratory capable
PIF	peak inspiratory flow
pMDI	pressurized metered dose inhaler
PRO	patient-reported outcome
RPM	remote patient monitoring
SABA	short-acting β-2 agonist
Vin	inhaled volume

REFERENCES

1. Chongmelaxme B, Chaiyakunapruk N, Dilokthornsakul P. Association between adherence and severe asthma exacerbation: A systematic review and meta-analysis. J Am Pharm Assoc 2020;60:669–685.
2. Price DB, Román-Rodríguez M, McQueen RB, et al. Inhaler errors in the CRITIKAL study: Type, frequency, and association with asthma outcomes. J Allergy Clin Immunol Pract 2017;5:1071–1081.
3. George M, Bender B. New insights to improve treatment adherence in asthma and COPD. Patient Prefer Adherence 2019;1:1325–1334.
4. George M. Adherence in asthma and COPD: New strategies for an old problem. Respir Care 2018;63:818–831.
5. Patel M, Perrin K, Pritchard A, et al. Accuracy of patient self-report as a measure of inhaled asthma medication use. Respirology 2013;3:546–552.
6. Pleasants RA, Hess DR. Aerosol delivery devices for obstructive lung diseases. Respir Care 2018;63:708–733.
7. Blakey JD, Bender BG, Dima AL, et al. Digital technologies and adherence in respiratory diseases: The road ahead. Eur Respir J 2018;52:1801147.
8. Chan AHY, Pleasants RA, Dhand R, et al. Digital inhalers for asthma or chronic obstructive pulmonary disease: A scientific perspective. Pulm Ther 2021;7:345–376.
9. Global digital dose inhalers market to reach $4.9 billion by 2026 – Benzinga. https://www.strategyr.com/market-report-digital-dose-inhalers-forecasts-global-industry-analysts-inc.asp
10. Mehta PP. Dry powder inhalers: A concise summary of the electronic monitoring devices. Ther Deliv 2021;1:1–6.
11. Janson C, Loof T, Telg G, et al. Impact of inhalation flow, inhalation volume and critical handling errors on delivered budesonide/formoterol dose in different inhalers: An in vitro study. Pulm Ther 2017;3:243–253.
12. Xiroudaki S, Schoubben A, Giovagnoli S, et al. Dry powder inhalers in the digitalization era: Current status and future perspectives. Pharmaceutics 2021;13:1455.
13. Dimitrova EK. Quality requirements for drug-device combinations. Available from: https://www.ema.europa.eu/en/quality-requirements-drug-device-combinations
14. Combination Products. [cited 2022 Apr 1]. Available from: https://www.fda.gov/media/114537/download
15. Guidance for the content of premarket submissions for software contained in medical devices. [cited 2022 Apr 1]. Available from: https://www.fda.gov/regulatory-information/search-fda-guidance-documents...
16. Policy for device software functions and mobile medical applications guidance for industry and food and drug administration staff. 2019. [cited 2022 Apr 1]. Available from: https://www.fda.gov/media/80958/download
17. Digital Health Center of Excellence | FDA. [cited 2022 Apr 1]. https://www.fda.gov/medical-devices/digital-health-center-excellence
18. https://www.fda.gov/about-fda/fda-organization/center-devices-and-radiological-health
19. Taitsman JK, Grimm CM, Argawal S. Protecting patient privacy and data security. N Engl J Med 2013;368:977–979.
20. Kim KK, Sankar P, Wilson MD, et al. Factors affecting willingness to share electronic health data among California consumers. BMC Med Ethics 2017;18:25.

21. Campbell JI, Eyal N, Musiimenta A, et al. Ethical questions in medical electronic adherence monitoring. J Gen Intern Med 2016;31(3):338–342.

22. Rockwern B, Johnson D, Sulmasy LS. Health information privacy, protection, and use in the expanding digital health ecosystem: A position paper of the American College of Physicians. Ann Intern Med 2021;174:994–998.

23. Foster JM, Smith L, Usherwood T, et al. The reliability and patient acceptability of the SmartTrack device: A new electronic monitor and reminder device for metered dose inhalers. J Asthma 2012;49:657–662.

24. Merchant R, Inamdar R, Henderson K, et al. Digital health intervention for asthma: Patient-reported value and usability. JMIR Mhealth Uhealth 2018;6(6):e133.

25. Sumino K, Locke ER, Magzamen S, et al. Use of a remote inhaler monitoring device to measure change in inhaler use with chronic obstructive pulmonary disease exacerbations. J Aerosol Med Pulm Drug Deliv 2018;31:191–198.

26. Chen J, Kaye L, Tuffli M, et al. Passive monitoring of short-acting beta-agonist use via digital platform in patient with chronic obstructive pulmonary disease: Quality improvement retrospective analysis. J Med Inform Res 2019;3:e13286.

27. Merchant RK, Inamdar R, Quade RC. Effectiveness of population health management using the propeller health asthma platform: A randomized clinical trial. J Allergy Clin Immunol Pract 2016;4:455–463.

28. Morton RW, Elphick HE, Rigby AS, et al. STAAR: A randomised controlled trial of electronic adherence monitoring with reminder alarms and feedback to improve clinical outcomes for children with asthma. Thorax 2017;72:347–354.

29. Lee J, Tay TR, Radhakrishna N, et al. Nonadherence in the era of severe asthma biologics and thermoplasty. Eur Respir J 2018;51:1701836.

30. Jochmann A, Artusio L, Jamalzadeh A, et al. Electronic monitoring of adherence to inhaled corticosteroids: An essential tool in identifying severe asthma in children. Eur Respir J 2017;50:1700910.

31. Moore A, Preece A, Sharma R, et al. A randomised controlled trial of the effect of a connected inhaler system on medication adherence in uncontrolled asthmatic patients. Eur Respir J 2021;57:2003103.

32. Mosnaim GS, Stempel DA, Gonzalez C, et al. The impact of patient self-monitoring via electronic medication monitor and mobile app plus remote clinician feedback on adherence to inhaled corticosteroids: A randomized controlled trial. J Allergy Clin Immunol Pract 2020;20:1586–1594.

33. O'Dwyer S, Greene G, MacHale E, et al. Personalized biofeedback on inhaler adherence and technique by community pharmacists: A cluster randomized clinical trial. J Allergy Clin Immunol Pract 2020;8(2):635–644.

34. Sulaiman I, Greene G, MacHale E, et al. A randomised clinical trial of feedback on inhaler adherence and technique in patients with severe uncontrolled asthma. Eur Respir J 2018;51:1701126.

35. Criner GJ, Cole T, Hahn KA, et al. The impact of budesonide/formoterol pMDI medication reminders on adherence in chronic obstructive pulmonary disease (COPD) patients: Results of a randomized, phase 4, clinical study. Int J Chron Obstruct Pulmon Dis 2021;16:563–577.

36. Bowler R, Allinder M, Jacobson S, et al. Real-world use of rescue inhaler sensors, electronic symptom questionnaires and physical activity monitors in COPD. BMJ Open Respir Res 2019;6(1):e000350.

37. Fan VS, Gylys-Colwell I, Locke E, et al. Overuse of short-acting betaagonist bronchodilators in COPD during periods of clinical stability. Respir Med 2016;116:100–106.
38. https://ginasthma.org/
39. Cloutier MM, Dixon AE, Krishnan JA, et al. Managing asthma in adolescents and adults: 2020 asthma guideline update from the National Asthma Education and Prevention Program. JAMA 2020;324:2301–2317.
40. https://goldcopd.org/2022-gold-reports-2
41. Patel M, Pilcher J, Reddel HK, et al. Metrics of salbutamol use as predictors of future adverse outcomes in asthma. Clin Exp Allergy 2013;43:1144–1151.
42. Pleasants R, Safioti G, Reich M, et al. Rescue medication use and inhalation patterns during asthma exacerbations recorded by Digihaler. Ann Allergy Asthma Immunol 2019;123:S14–S17.
43. Snyder LD, Safioti G, Reich M, et al. Objective assessment of rescue medication use and inhalation characteristics of COPD patients recorded by the electronic ProAir Digihaler. Am J Respir Crit Care Med 2020;201:A4305.
44. Tashkin DP. A review of nebulized drug delivery in COPD. Int J Chron Obstruct Pulmon Dis 2016;11:2585–2596.
45. Lacasse Y, Archibald H, Ernst P, et al. Patterns and determinants of compliance with inhaled steroids in adults with asthma. Can Respir J 2005;12:211–217.
46. Tibble H, Chan A, Mitchell EA, et al. A data-driven typology of asthma medication adherence using cluster analysis. Sci Rep 2020;10(1):1–8.
47. Sulaiman I, Cushen B, Greene G, et al. Objective assessment of adherence to inhalers by patients with chronic obstructive pulmonary disease. Am J Respir Crit Care Med 2017;195:1333–1343.
48. De Keyser HEH, Kaye L, Anderson WC, et al. Electronic medication monitors help determine adherence subgroups in asthma. Respir Med 2020;164:105914.
49. Sulaiman I, Seheult J, MacHale E, et al. Irregular and ineffective: A quantitative observational study of the time and technique of inhaler use. J Allergy Clin Immunol Pract 2016;4:900–909.
50. Normansell R, Kew KM, Stovold E. Interventions to improve adherence to inhaled steroids for asthma. Cochrane Database Syst Rev 2017;4:CD012226.
51. Mueller S, Wilke T, Bechtel B, et al. Non-persistence and non-adherence to long-acting COPD medication therapy: A retrospective cohort study based on a large German claims dataset. Respir Med 2017;122:1–11.
52. Killane I, Sulaiman I, MacHale E, et al. Predicting asthma exacerbations employing remotely monitored adherence. Healthc Technol Lett 2016;3:51–55.
53. Vestbo J, Anderson, Calverley JP, et al. Adherence to inhaled therapy, mortality and hospital admission in COPD. Thorax 2009;64:939–943.
54. Dekhuijzen R, Lavorini F, Usmani OS, et al. Addressing the impact and unmet needs of nonadherence in asthma and chronic obstructive pulmonary disease: Where do we go from here? J Allergy Clin Immunol Pract 2018;6:785–793.
55. Jackson DJ, Bacharier LB. Inhaled corticosteroids for the prevention of asthma exacerbations. Ann Allergy Asthma Immunol 2021;127:524–529.
56. Chan AH, Stewart AW, Harrison J, et al. The effect of an electronic monitoring device with audiovisual reminder function on adherence to inhaled corticosteroids and school attendance in children with asthma: A randomised controlled trial. Lancet Respir Med 2015;3:210–219.

57. Foster JM, Usherwood T, Smith L, et al. Inhaler reminders improve adherence with controller treatment in primary care patients with asthma. J Allergy Clin Immunol 2014;134:1260–1268.

58. Gregoriano C, Dieterle T, Breitenstein AL, et al. Does a tailored intervention to promote adherence in patients with chronic lung disease affect exacerbations? A randomized controlled trial. Respir Res 2019;20:273.

59. Patel M, Pilcher J, Pritchard A, et al. Efficacy and safety of maintenance and reliever combination budesonide–formoterol inhaler in patients with asthma at risk of severe exacerbations: A randomised controlled trial. Lancet Respir Med 2013;1:32–42.

60. Broeders MEAC, Molema J, Hop WCJ, et al. The course of inhalation profiles during an exacerbation of obstructive lung disease. Respir Med 2004;98:1173–1179.

61. Taube C, Kanniess F, Grönke L, et al. Reproducibility of forced inspiratory and expiratory volumes after bronchodilation in patients with COPD or asthma. Respir Med 2003;97:568–577.

62. O'Donnell DE, Forkert L, Webb KA. Evaluation of bronchodilator responses in patients with "irreversible" emphysema. Eur Respir J 2001;18:914–920.

63. Bass H. The flow volume loop: Normal standards and abnormalities in chronic obstructive pulmonary disease. Chest 1973;63:171–175.

64. Wells RE. Mechanics of respiration in bronchial asthma. Am J Med 1959;384–393.

65. Chrystyn H, Soussi M, Tarsin W, et al. Inhalation characteristics when patients use a dry powder inhaler (DPI) are related to their lung function when they are stable and when recovering from an acute exacerbations. Am J Respir Crit Care Med 2020;201:A3939.

66. Watz H, Tetzlaff K, Magnussen H, et al. Spirometric changes during exacerbations of COPD: A post hoc analysis of the WISDOM trial. Respir Res 2018;19:251.

67. Chrystyn H, Saralaya D, Shenoy A, et al. Investigating the accuracy of the Digihaler, a new electronic multidose dry-powder inhaler, in measuring inhalation parameters. J Aerosol Med Pulm Drug Deliv 2022;35:166–177. DOI:10.1089/jamp.2021.0031

68. D'Arcy S, MacHale E, Seheult J, et al. A method to assess adherence in inhaler use through analysis of acoustic recordings of inhaler events. PLoS One 2014;9(6):e98701.

69. Rogueda P, Grinovero M, Ponti L, et al. Telehealth ready: Performance of the Amiko Respiro Sense connected technology with Merxin DPIs. Drug Delivery to the Lungs (DDL2018).

70. Pilcher J, Shirtcliffe P, Patel M, et al. Three-month validation of a turbuhaler electronic monitoring device: Implications for asthma clinical trial use. BMJ Open Respir Res 2015;2:e000097.

71. Patel M, Pilcher J, Chan A, et al. Six-month in vitro validation of a metered-dose inhaler electronic monitoring device: Implications for asthma clinical trial use. J Allergy Clin Immunol 2012;130:1420–1422.

72. Mokoka MC, McDonnell MJ, MacHale E, et al. Inadequate assessment of adherence to maintenance medication leads to loss of power and increased costs in trials of severe asthma therapy: Results from a systematic literature review and modelling study. Eur Respir J.2019;53(5):1802161.

73. Jochmann A, Artusio L, Usemann J, et al. A 3-month period of electronic monitoring can provide important information to the healthcare team to assess adherence and improve asthma control. ERJ Open Res 2021;7.

8 Nebulizers

Paul D. Terry and Rajiv Dhand

CONTENTS

INTRODUCTION

Nebulizers convert liquid medicines into a fine mist for inhalation, typically to treat a variety of airway disorders, such as asthma, chronic obstructive pulmonary disease (COPD), and cystic fibrosis (CF). Nebulizers are commonly used for rescue therapy to provide rapid short-term relief of acute respiratory conditions, such as acute exacerbations of asthma, COPD, and acute bronchospasm. When first developed in the mid-nineteenth century, nebulizers used hand-held pumps to force a liquid against a plate or baffle, nebulizing (or "atomizing") it for inhalation through a tube or mask. For example, "the Pulverisateur," invented in France in 1858, was a large, heavy, and cumbersome device that used a bicycle-style pump to draw solution from a glass reservoir and force it through a small nozzle into an impaction plate to produce an inhalable mist (1). The first electric nebulizers, invented in Europe in the early 1930s, used compressed air to nebulize a variety of medicines thought to improve asthma symptoms (2). An early example was the "Pneumostat," invented in Germany in the early 1930s, a large, noisy, nine-pound device that was affordable to own only to the very wealthy (1). Over time, incremental improvements were made in nebulizers to maximize drug penetration into the lungs. Today's nebulizers are small, light, quiet, and are often battery-operated, making them increasingly portable and convenient to use.

Three types of nebulizer designs are commonly used in clinical practice, namely, jet or pneumatic nebulizers, ultrasonic nebulizers, and vibrating mesh nebulizers.

DOI: 10.1201/9781003269014-8

JET NEBULIZERS

Jet, or pneumatic, nebulizers use compressed air or oxygen to draw liquid from a reservoir and nebulize it into droplets against internal baffles (Figure 8.1). By forcing air through a constricted outlet to increase its velocity, the nebulizer creates a vacuum that pulls medicine up a capillary tube into the "jet stream," hence the name. Most modern jet nebulizers are powered by high-pressure air or oxygen provided by a tabletop compressor, compressed gas cylinder, or 50-psi wall outlet. Patients typically receive nebulizer therapy through small-volume nebulizer units (capacity 5–20 mL), but some receive large-volume nebulizer therapy (capacity up to 200 mL) for longer-term treatment, or "In-line" therapy when operated in a ventilator circuit.

Typical nebulizer equipment consists of a pressurized gas source, a flowmeter, oxygen tubing, a medicine cup, a mouthpiece or mask, a normal saline solution, and the prescribed medication. The treatment time for jet nebulizers ranges between 10 and 25 minutes (3), depending on the airflow rate used to drive the nebulizer. The driving pressure or the flow rate of compressed air applied to the jet affects aerosol output and particle size from jet nebulizers. The higher the pressure or flow rate, the greater the output over time in terms of the total solution aerosolized, and the smaller the particle size (3). A gas flow of 6 to 8 L/min is usually selected to optimize drug delivery (4). The mass median aerodynamic diameter (MMAD) of aerosols produced by jet

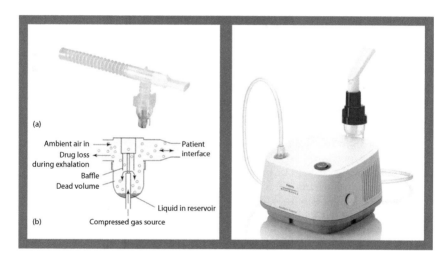

Figure 8.1 The left panel shows components of a jet nebulizer (a). In (b), the operation of jet nebulizers is shown. Compressed gas is delivered through a jet, and the expansion of the jet creates a negative pressure that entrains the solution to be aerosolized into the gas stream. The solution is sheared into a liquid film that is unstable and breaks into droplets because of surface tension forces. A baffle is placed in the aerosol stream and the larger particles impact the baffle and are returned to the nebulizer reservoir, whereas the smaller particles are carried by the airstream to the patient. The right panel shows the components of a jet nebulizer for home use including a nebulizer, mouthpiece (or facemask), connecting tubing, and compressor unit.

nebulizers varies but should be between 1 and 4 μm to optimize deposition in the lower respiratory tract. The density of the gas powering the nebulizer also affects nebulizer performance. In the rare situation that the nebulizer is powered with heliox (helium:oxygen 80:20), the gas flow to the nebulizer is increased by at least 50% to 9–15 L/min to compensate for the lower density of the gas (5).

Jet nebulizers are not inherently efficient for drug delivery to the lung. Significant amounts of aerosolized medicine can be trapped within the nebulizer, in the connecting T-piece and in the mouthpiece or face mask. As a result of the continuous aerosol output during treatment, much of the medicine can also be lost to the atmosphere during exhalation (3). The high flow of gas through a jet nebulizer evaporates solvent during nebulization and adiabatic expansion of the gas cools the output air and concentrates the solution in the nebulizer cup. The rate of evaporation depends on the volume of fluid placed in the reservoir. Nebulizer output can cool by >10°C below ambient temperature during treatment and the concentration of the reservoir solution can increase by up to 30% (6, 7). With a reservoir fill volume of 3 to 5 mL, compared with the 2 mL in the unit dose "nebules," a greater total amount of drug is aerosolized and delivered to the patient, albeit with a longer treatment time (3, 8). At the end of nebulization, when no further aerosol is produced, ~0.5–1.5 mL of the concentrated solution remains in the nebulizer reservoir as a *dead volume* containing drug that is unavailable to the patient (3, 8). Some common terms are used to describe the "dose" of the drug delivered by nebulizers (Table 8.1).

Jet nebulizers are the most employed nebulizers in clinical practice because they are reliable, durable, and economical, but they are not inherently a quiet or highly efficient design and are not always conveniently small. Jet nebulizers have inherent advantages and disadvantages, and variances in nebulizer performance are a function not only of their design but also of the source of energy (compressed gas or electrical compressor), gas flow and pressure, connecting tubing, interface used (spacer, and mouthpiece or mask), and the patient's breathing pattern (9). The interplay of these factors results in significant variations in nebulizer performance not only among different brands but also between nebulizers of the same brand (10–12). Other factors that influence nebulizer performance include the viscosity, density, and surface tension of the solution to be nebulized. Increasing the viscosity of the solution, such as with increasing concentrations of some medications, could decrease the nebulizer output rate as well as droplet size (13, 14). In contrast, reducing the surface tension increases nebulizer output (15). When suspensions, instead of solutions, are nebulized in a jet nebulizer, the aerosol droplets are larger compared to those with solution formulations (16).

Technological improvements that have accrued in jet nebulizers over time include conventional constant-output models with a corrugated tube acting as a reservoir, which increases efficiency by mitigating drug loss, particularly during exhalation (12). In jet nebulizers with a collection bag, aerosol generated during expiration is stored in the collection bag and is available to the patient with the next inspiration. A one-way valve located between the mouthpiece and the nebulizer separates fresh gas from exhaled gas (12). To further address the aerosol delivery inefficiencies, newer designs, such as breath-enhanced jet nebulizers, release more aerosol during inhalation, whereas breath-actuated jet nebulizers sense the patient's inspiratory flow and deliver aerosol only on inspiration, with consequent less wastage of drug

Table 8.1: **Nebulizer Dose, Lung Aerosol Deposition, and Drug Effects**

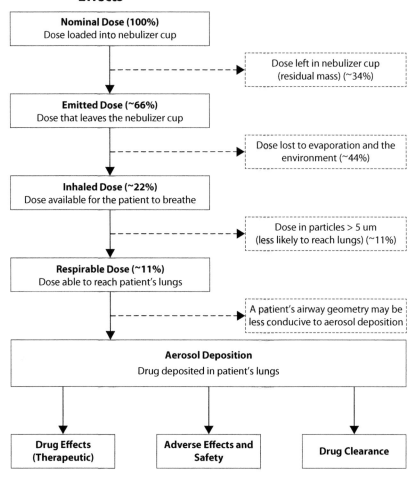

(Figure 8.2). In breath-enhanced nebulizers, for example, the PARI LC Plus (Starnberg, Germany), additional airflow is routed through the nebulizer during inspiration to enhance aerosol generation, and in some designs, one-way valves are provided to reduce aerosol output during exhalation (17–19). In a dosimetric nebulizer, either manual interruption of airflow, as in the Pari LL, or by a spring-loaded valve, as in the AeroEclipse, prevents aerosol generation during exhalation. The AeroEclipse has a higher output than a breath-enhanced nebulizer (PARI LCD, Starnberg, Germany) (20).

Large-volume nebulizers, such as the high-output extended aerosol respiratory therapy (HEART) nebulizer (Cardinal Health, Dublin, OH, US), Air Life Misty Finity (Vyaire, Chicago, IL, US), Flo-Mist (Smiths Medical, Minneapolis, MN, US) and HOPE nebulizer (B&B Medical Technologies, Carlsbad, CA, US) have reservoirs larger than 200 mL and are designed for continuous aerosol delivery (see below).

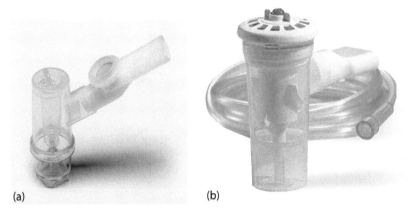

(a)   (b)

Figure 8.2   Examples of breath-enhanced (a) and breath-actuated nebulizers (b). In the breath-enhanced nebulizer (Nebutech, Salter Labs, Hudson, NH, US), the patient breathes through the nebulizer during inspiration, thereby increasing airflow and enhancing nebulizer output. During exhalation, a one-way valve directs away from the nebulizer chamber and aerosol output is decreased. In the breath-actuated nebulizer (AeroEclipse, Monaghan, Plattsburgh, NY, US), a breath-actuated valve allows airflow only during inhalation so that no aerosol is produced during exhalation and aerosol loss is minimized.

ULTRASONIC NEBULIZERS

Ultrasonic atomization, first used in humidifiers, was adapted for nebulizer use in the mid-1960s, an innovation that allowed the production of finer aerosols than were typical of jet nebulizers at that time, in smaller, quieter devices, and with shorter durations of treatment (Figure 8.3) (2, 21). These devices transmit sound waves generated by vibrating a piezoelectric crystal at high frequency (~1–3 MHz) to the surface of the drug solution, generating aerosol that is typically more consistent in size than that produced by jet nebulizers (22–24). The size of the particles generated by ultrasonic nebulizers is inversely proportional to the vibration frequency of the piezo crystal. The surface tension and density of the solution also influence droplet size (25). Compared with jet nebulizers, most ultrasonic nebulizers have a faster rate of nebulization, require a shorter operation time, and have a larger aerosol particle size (26). The particle size and aerosol density produced by ultrasonic nebulizers also depend on the gas flow carrying the aerosol particles from the nebulizer to the patient. The increase in solution concentration during ultrasonic nebulizer operation is less pronounced than with jet nebulizers (27). Unlike jet nebulizers, the solution temperature increases by 10°C to 15°C after 10 minutes of ultrasonic nebulization (27), and this could denature thermolabile therapeutic agents.

The cost and bulk of ultrasonic nebulizers, their tendency for mechanical malfunction, and their relative inefficiency in nebulizing drug suspensions (28), liposomes (29), or more viscous solutions, are major limitations to their use. Hence, ultrasonic nebulizers are less commonly used than other nebulizer designs. Several small-volume ultrasonic nebulizers (Beetle Neb, Drive Medical, Chicago, IL, US; Lumiscope, Just Nebulizers, Fulton, MD, US; Minibreeze, Mabis DMI, Ontario, Canada) in which drug solutions, including bronchodilators,

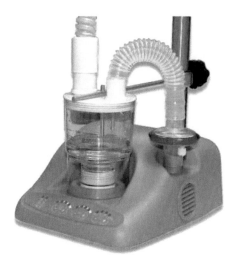

Figure 8.3 Illustration showing a high throughput ultrasonic nebulizer that can be used for humidification or inhalation therapy (DeVilbiss ultrasonic nebulizer, Somerset, PA). The unit can be wall mounted with a rail clamp or placed on a movable stand for greater flexibility. The integrated timer features settings of 0/15/30/45 or 60 minutes.

anti-inflammatory agents, and antibiotics, are placed directly into the manifold on top of the transducer, have been marketed to improve portability. These devices use the patient's inspiratory airflow to carry the aerosol from the nebulizer.

VIBRATING MESH NEBULIZERS

Mesh technology emerged in nebulizer devices in the 1980s and 1990s (30, 31). Like ultrasonic nebulizers, active mesh nebulizers, such as the Aerogen (Galway, Ireland) or eFlow nebulizers (PARI, Starnberg, Germany), use energy from a vibrating piezoelectric element to mechanically pump the solution through a vibrating membrane ("mesh") at the top of the liquid reservoir (Figure 8.4) (32). A dome-shaped aperture plate is attached to a plate that is connected to a piezo-ceramic element surrounding the aperture plate. When energy is applied to the piezoelectric element, the aperture plate vibrates at ~130 kHz. The up and down movement of the plate, by about 1 µm, creates a micro-pumping action, whereby short filaments of the solution liquid pass through 1000–7000 laser-drilled holes in the aperture plate and break up into droplets that are overall finer, and more consistent in particle size than those produced by ultrasonic nebulizers. The size of the droplets depends on several factors, including the shape and size of the holes in the mesh, and the surface tension and viscosity of the solution. In contrast with jet nebulizers, vibrating mesh nebulizers have smaller residual volumes (ranging from 0.1 to 0.4 mL); the nebulizer drug output is higher, and the exit velocity of the aerosol is lower (<4 m/s).

In passive vibrating mesh nebulizers, such as the MicroAir U100 (Omron, Kyoto, Japan) or I-neb (Philips Respironics, Murrysville, PA, US), the mesh

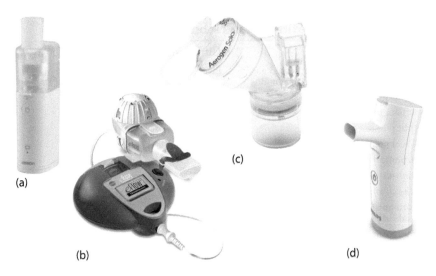

Figure 8.4 Examples of vibrating mesh nebulizers, including the Omron NE-U100 portable MicroAir (a); PARI eFlow (b), Aerogen Solo (c), and Philips Innospire Go (d).

is separated from an ultrasonic horn by the solution to be nebulized. A piezoelectric transducer vibrates the horn and the vibrations of the horn push the solution through the mesh (32).

Mesh nebulizers have shorter treatment times of ~5–7 minutes, with less undesired heating or waste of the liquid than previous designs, all in smaller, more portable, quieter, battery-operated devices (12, 31) (Table 8.2). For example, the InnoSpire Go mesh nebulizer (Figure 8.4) delivers treatment in a small, light (111 g), quiet (<35 dB), upright design that can be filled and used up to 30 times from a single charge of the internal battery, without removable parts that require manipulation. Thus, mesh nebulizers may be preferred over compressor-driven jet nebulizers for their convenience, ease of use, and treatment satisfaction (33). Moreover, suspension formulations, such as budesonide, and various antibiotics can be delivered by mesh nebulizers, although viscous drugs and suspensions can clog the mesh's pores (12, 30). For these reasons, vibrating mesh nebulizers are convenient for use in outpatients and during the mechanical ventilation of hospitalized patients (34). The higher efficiency of the vibrating mesh nebulizers to deliver drugs to the lungs could result in greater systemic side effects, hence the nominal dose of the drug may need to be adjusted according to the efficiency of the delivery system (34).

The vibrating mesh technology has been adapted for volumetric nebulization, whereby the drug solution is dripped from a tube feed and pump system directly onto the surface of the mesh. The rate of nebulization is determined by the output of the solution by the syringe pump, and the infusion rate should not exceed the maximum output rate of the mesh. Some mesh nebulizers can aerosolize single drops (~15 µL) of various formulations.

Despite its advantages, vibrating mesh technology is expensive to manufacture and comes with a significantly increased cost for the consumer, particularly compared with jet nebulizers (Table 8.2). Mesh nebulizers must also

Table 8.2: Comparison of Characteristics of Jet, Ultrasonic, and Vibrating Mesh Nebulizers

Features	Jet	Ultrasonic	Vibrating Mesh
Power source	Compressed gas/ electrical mains	Electrical mains	Batteries/electrical mains
Portability	Limited	Limited	Portable
Treatment time	Long	Intermediate	Short
Output rate	Low	Higher	Highest
Residual volume	0.5–1.5 mL	Variable but low	≤ 0.2 mL
Environmental Contamination			
Continuous use	High	High	High
Breath-activated	Low	Low	Low
Performance Variability	High	Intermediate	Low
Formulation Characteristics			
Concentration	Increases	Variable	No change
Temperature	Decreases	Increases	Minimal change
Suspensions	Low efficiency	Poor efficiency	Variable
Denaturation	Possible[a]	Probable[a]	Possible[a]
Cleaning	Required	Required	Required
	Single-patient use	Multiple-patient use	Single-patient use
Cost	Very low	High	High

[a] Denaturation of DNA occurs with all the nebulizers.

be cleaned regularly to prevent buildup and blockage of the mesh apertures, especially when drug suspensions are aerosolized.

ADAPTIVE AEROSOL DELIVERY (AAD)

The products of new technologies include "intelligent" nebulizers such as the I-neb Adaptive Aerosol Delivery (AAD) System for the delivery of prostacyclin (12). The I-neb AAD System continuously adapts to changes in the patient's breathing pattern and pulses aerosol only during the inspiratory part of the breathing cycle (35). This eliminates the waste of aerosol during exhalation and provides precise aerosol dose delivery from a unique metering chamber design. Through the vibrating mesh technology, the metering chamber design, and the AAD Disc function, the aerosol output rate and metered dose can be tailored to the demands of the specific drug to be delivered. In the I-neb AAD System, aerosol delivery is guided through two algorithms, one for the Tidal Breathing Mode (TBM), and one for slow and deep inhalations, the Target Inhalation Mode (TIM). The aim of TIM is to reduce the treatment time by increasing the total inhalation time per minute and to increase lung deposition by reducing impaction in the upper airways through slow and deep inhalations. A key feature of the AAD technology is the patient feedback mechanisms that guide the patient on delivery performance and signal completion of the dose. These feedback signals, which include visual, audible, and tactile forms, appear to promote a high level of compliance with the use of the I-neb AAD System (Philips Respironics, Murrysville, PA) (35).

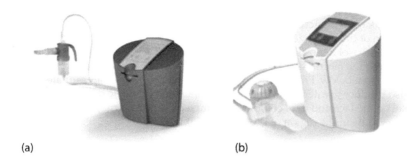

(a)   (b)

Figure 8.5 The AKITA jet nebulizer system (left panel) and the AKITA 2 system (right panel) are shown (Vectura Delivery Devices, Cambridge, UK). The AKITA 2 system uses the PARI APIXNEB vibrating mesh nebulizer.

AKITA SYSTEM

The AKITA device (Vectura Delivery Devices, Cambridge, UK) applies positive pressure delivered with a computer-controlled compressor to control the entire inhalation maneuver of the patient (Figure 8.5). It has been used with both conventional jet nebulizers and vibrating mesh nebulizers. The AKITA system improves delivery efficiency (36), with up to 60% drug deposition in the lung periphery of patients with COPD, and >80% pulmonary deposition in CF patients (37). The device stores the patient's pulmonary function on a smart card that is programmed to generate aerosol during specific phases of inspiration. Aerosol generation during early inspiration targets more peripheral airways, whereas central airways could be targeted by aerosol generation during the later phases of inspiration (38). The AKITA 2 system uses the PARI APIXNEB vibrating mesh nebulizer (Figure 8.5), and its use in patients with asthma for targeting small airways with high-dose inhaled corticosteroids reduced the number of exacerbations requiring oral corticosteroids over one year of treatment (39).

SMALL PARTICLE AEROSOL GENERATOR (SPAG)

The small particle aerosol generator (SPAG; ICN Pharmaceuticals, Costa Mesa, CA), a large-volume, pneumatically powered nebulizer, is used to aerosolize Ribavirin. It employs a drying chamber with its own flow control to produce an extra fine aerosol (MMAD 1.2–1.4 μm) with a relatively high output. In mechanically ventilated infants with severe Respiratory Syncytial Virus (RSV) infection, aerosol administration of Ribavirin with SPAG reduced the duration of ventilation, oxygen support, and hospital stay (40).

EFFECT OF FORMULATION

The presence of a preservative in a drug solution and admixture with other drugs affect nebulizer output and aerosol characteristics (15, 41, 42). Drug mixtures need to be physically and chemically compatible (43–46).

MOUTHPIECE VERSUS FACEMASK DELIVERY

Aerosol deposition in nasal passages significantly reduces drug delivery to the lung (47–49) and could reduce bronchodilator efficacy when the nebulizer is employed with a facemask versus a mouthpiece (50). Facemasks may be necessary for the treatment of acutely dyspneic or uncooperative patients. For optimal efficacy, the facemask should produce a tight seal (51–53) to avoid aerosol leakage and increased aerosol deposition around the eyes (54). The orientation of the nebulizer with respect to the facemask also influences the pattern of aerosol deposition. In "Front-loaded" masks, the nebulizer is inserted directly into the facemask, whereas in "Bottom-loaded" masks the aerosol enters the mask from below. Front-loaded masks provide not only greater inhaled mass but also produce greater facial and ocular deposition (55). The deposition of aerosol on the face and eyes could be minimized by using a mask with vents, as well as cutouts in the region of the eyes (55, 56).

CONTINUOUS AEROSOL DELIVERY

In patients with acute severe asthma, short-acting bronchodilators (e.g., albuterol 5–15 mg/h) (57) are often given continuously. Large-volume nebulizers or the HEART nebulizer are commonly used for continuous aerosol delivery because they can provide consistent drug output for 4–8 h, respectively (58–60). A Cochrane Review found that patients with acute asthma derive modest benefits from continuous bronchodilator therapy in the Emergency Room setting (61). Solutions in large-volume nebulizers may become increasingly concentrated over several hours of use and patients need close monitoring for signs of drug toxicity (59).

NEBULIZER USE IN THE TIME OF COVID-19

Aerosol that does not deposit in the lung during a patient's inhalation can exit a nebulizer into the ambient environment during exhalation. Therefore, there is concern about the potential risk for transmission of severe acute respiratory syndrome coronavirus 2 (SARS-CoV-2) through aerosolized respiratory droplets during the treatment of patients with coronavirus disease 19 (COVID-19) (62). Due to concerns that aerosol generated by the nebulizer might carry the virus to the surrounding environment, several clinical societies made recommendations against the use of nebulizers during the COVID-19 pandemic (63, 64). However, there is currently no conclusive evidence supporting an increased risk of viral transmission during nebulization in COVID-19 patients, or for patients to switch to treatment via hand-held inhalers for the reason of preventing infection. Jain and coworkers performed a pilot clinical study using scintigraphy to investigate the dispersion pattern of technetium (Tc)-radiolabeled exhaled droplets during nebulization with a jet nebulizer and compressor (65). The authors reported that nebulizer use did not affect the dispersion of respiratory aerosols during tidal breathing. These results suggest that nebulization *per se* has a clinically insignificant role in the dispersion of exhaled aerosols. Consistent with this view, guidelines from other expert groups, such as The National Institute for Health and Care Excellence (NICE) in the UK, The New and Emerging Respiratory Virus Threats Advisory Group (NERVTAG) (66–68), and The Centers for Disease Control and Prevention (CDC) in the US (69), have not advised against the use of nebulizers during the COVID pandemic.

There are several ways to mitigate even a small risk of virus transmission during nebulizer therapy. The type of nebulizer device, type of interface, flow rate, and patient characteristics can affect fugitive emissions during nebulizer treatment. For example, McGrath et al. (70) used a simulation model to show higher fugitive aerosol concentrations with tracheostomy interfaces compared with those from nasal cannula when using pediatric, but not adult, breathing profiles. The study also found that as the flow rate increased, fugitive emissions and MMAD of the aerosol both decreased. Another simulation by Avari et al. (71)

compared viral dispersion (nebulized bacteriophages) from several respiratory support methods, finding the highest air concentrations with the use of high-flow nasal oxygen and nasal prongs, and the lowest concentrations with the use of invasive ventilation and helmet ventilation with a positive end-expiratory pressure (PEEP) valve. Li and colleagues provide guidance for reducing fugitive aerosol emissions from nebulizers in clinical practice (72). They conducted a study on nine healthy volunteers who were given saline with a small-volume nebulizer (SVN) or vibrating mesh nebulizer (VMN). They found that SVN produced higher fugitive aerosol concentrations than VMN, whereas facemasks generated higher aerosol concentrations than mouthpieces. Adding an exhalation filter to the mouthpiece or a scavenger to the facemask reduced fugitive aerosol concentrations for both SVN and VMN (72).

Notwithstanding the nebulizer type used, the medication loading process needs to be performed using an aseptic technique to prevent contamination of the reservoir and reduce the risk of bio-aerosol dispersion. A mouthpiece should be preferred over a facemask to improve treatment efficiency and reduce fugitive emissions (70). Furthermore, placing a filter on the nebulizer's outlet reduces exposure of health care personnel (HCP) to aerosol medications (72–74). An exhalation filter attached to a jet nebulizer reduced exhaled aerosol droplets between 0.06 and 0.1 μm in size by 98% (75). Thus, the emission of exhaled aerosol droplets from jet or mesh nebulizers could be effectively reduced by use of a mouthpiece and a filter attached to the exhalation port of the nebulizer. In hospital settings, the use of appropriate Personal Protective Equipment (PPE) by HCP, including N-95 mask, face shield, gloves, and gown, as well as powered air-purifying respirators (PAPRs) if needed, can also reduce transmission of infectious agents during nebulizer use (76).

INSTRUCTIONS FOR GENERAL NEBULIZER USE

What follows are basic guidelines for nebulizer use. However, consumers should always carefully read and understand the manufacturer's instructions. Nebulizers could be operated by a gas source of 50 psi from a wall source or compressed gas from a cylinder. When nebulizers are used at home, they are generally operated by gas flow from a compressor that provides a lower pressure. Nebulizers used for home care must be matched to an appropriate compressor to ensure optimal particle sizes and adequate drug output in the emitted aerosol (77).

- Wash hands with soap and water before preparing the nebulizer for use.

- Place the machine on a hard surface. Check to see if the air filter in the compressor is clean. If it is dirty, rinse it using cold water and let it air dry. Plug in the machine.

- With premixed medicine, open the medicine container and place the medication in the nebulizer cup. If medicines need to be mixed, place the correct amounts into the container using a dropper or syringe.

- Add sterile normal saline if needed.

- Connect the medicine container to the machine using the tubing. Connect the mask or mouthpiece to the top of the container.

- Place the mouthpiece between your teeth. Close your lips around it. When using a mask, place the mask on your face.

- Turn on the machine. Keep the medicine container in an upright position. Breathe in and out slowly and deeply through your mouth until the mist is gone.

- The treatment is over when all the medicine is gone or there is no more mist coming out. The treatment should be stopped when the nebulizer begins to sputter (78). The entire treatment may take up to 20 minutes.

GENERAL NEBULIZER CLEANING
Jet Nebulizers

To start, remove the tubing and set it aside. Never place the compressor under water.

After Each Use

i. Disassemble the nebulizer and discard any remaining solution from the medication cup.

ii. Rinse each piece under warm running water for 30 seconds.

iii. Tap out excess water and lay pieces on a lint-free cloth to dry.

iv. Store the plastic tubing and medication chamber in a plastic bag between uses.

At the End of Each Day

i. Disassemble the nebulizer and discard any remaining solution from the medication cup.

ii. Leave each piece submerged in a bowl of warm, soapy water for 30 minutes.

iii. Rinse each piece under warm water for 30 seconds.

iv. Tap out excess water and lay pieces on a lint-free cloth to dry.

v. Change the nebulizer daily when appropriate for infectious disease control, such as with COVID-19.

Disinfect Every 3 Days

i. Disassemble nebulizer.

ii. Place all pieces in a large bowl with two parts of sterile water and one part of white vinegar, fully submerged, for 30–60 minutes, or with a dilute solution of a quaternary ammonium compound, such as benzalkonium chloride, for 10 minutes, or per the manufacturer's instructions.

iii. Rinse each piece under warm water for 30 seconds.

iv. Tap out excess water and lay pieces on a lint-free cloth and dry overnight.

v. Clean the outside surface of the nebulizer with cloth soaked with 70% alcohol.

Longer Term

Most compressors have an air filter that needs to be replaced every 6 months and/or per the manufacturer's instructions.

Table 8.3: Cleaning Instructions for Four Commonly Used Vibrating Mesh Nebulizers

Mesh Nebulizer	Link to Cleaning Instructions
InnoSpire Go (Philips)	https://www.healthstore.philips.com/cleaning
Aerogen Solo / Aerogen Pro (Aerogen)	https://www.aerogen.com/wp-content/uploads/2017/05/30-914-Rev-D-Aerogen-USB-Controller-IM-US-WEB.pdf (pp. 25-29)
Pari eFlow Nebulizer System (Pari)	https://www.manualslib.com/manual/1618550/Pari-Eflow-Rapid-178g1005.html?page=46
Akita Jet Nebulizer (Vectura)	https://www.manualslib.com/manual/1732099/Vectura-Akita-Jet.html?page=12#manual

Vibrating Mesh Nebulizers

Cleaning instructions for vibrating mesh nebulizers are generally similar to those for jet nebulizers but can be more idiosyncratic depending on the brand. Most models require disassembly, rinsing, and cleaning of individual parts after each use, disinfection daily (which may include boiling or use of disinfection solution), and unclogging the aerosol head as needed. However, some require additional nebulization of cleaning or disinfection solution or distilled water; in this regard, some models have their own self-cleaning program. Here, we provide website links to cleaning instructions for a few commonly used vibrating mesh nebulizers (Table 8.3).

Multi-dose drug solutions for use in nebulizers have the potential to become contaminated. This can be prevented by refrigerating the solutions and discarding the syringes every 24 h (79, 80).

ADVANTAGES AND DISADVANTAGES OF NEBULIZERS

Nebulizers have several advantages and disadvantages when compared with other inhalation devices, namely pressurized metered dose inhalers (pMDIs), dry powder inhalers (DPIs), and soft mist inhalers (SMIs) (81) (Table 8.4). Some advantages of nebulizers are related to the technique and training required to use the device, convenience, capacity to deliver a higher drug dose, ability to aerosolize solutions and suspensions, including medications that are not available for aerosolization with inhalers, and several other considerations (Table 8.4).

Technique and Ease of Use

Nebulizers can be used by patients of any age and are commonly used to deliver medicine to children. Because the nebulizer treatments last several minutes and there is no need for training on a specific breathing pattern, nebulizers are more forgiving of faulty technique compared to inhalers. Indeed, inhaler use, particularly in elderly patients, is subject to several critical and non-critical errors that result in inadequate symptom relief for patients (82, 83). However, nebulizers are not free of potential problems with their use. For example, basic nebulizer inhalation technique, such as sitting in an upright position during therapy, may not be practiced by all patients (84).

Table 8.4: Advantages and Disadvantages of Each Type of Aerosol-Generating Device or System Clinically Available

Type	Advantages	Disadvantages
Small-Volume Jet Nebulizer	Patient coordination not required	Lack of portability
	Effective with tidal breathing	Pressurized gas source required
	High dose possible	Lengthy treatment time
	Dose modification possible	Device cleaning required
	No HFA release	Contamination possible
	Can be used with supplemental oxygen	Not all medications available in solution form
	Can deliver combination therapies if compatible	Does not aerosolize suspensions well
	Able to deliver solutions of drugs (e.g., dornase alfa) not available in other devices	Device preparation required
		Performance variability
		Expensive when compressor is added in
Ultrasonic Nebulizer	Patient coordination not required	Expensive
	High dose possible	Need for electrical power source (wall outlet or batteries)
	Dose modification possible	Contamination possible
	No HFA release	Not all medications available in solution form
	Small dead volume	Device preparation required before treatment
	Quiet	Does not nebulize suspensions well
	Newer designs small and portable	Possible drug degradation
	Faster delivery than jet nebulizer	Potential for airway irritation with some drugs
Vibrating Mesh	No drug loss during exhalation (breath-actuated devices)	Frequent malfunctions
	Small and portable	Relatively expensive
	Quiet operation	Difficulty delivering viscous drugs and suspensions
	Reduced treatment times	Can be difficult to clean
	Increased output volume and efficiency	
	Consistent fine-particle generation	
	Higher drug deposition in the lungs	
	Output rate adjustable	
	Can work with low drug volumes	
	Low residual volumes	
	Not likely to overheat drug solutions	

(Continued)

Table 8.4: Advantages and Disadvantages of Each Type of Aerosol-Generating Device or System Clinically Available *(Continued)*

Type	Advantages	Disadvantages
Pressurized MDI	Portable and compact	Coordination of breathing and actuation needed
	Treatment time is short	Device actuation required
	No drug preparation required	High pharyngeal deposition
	No contamination of contents	Upper limit to unit dose content
	Dose-dose reproducibility high	Potential for abuse
	Some can be used with breath-actuated mouthpiece	
		Not all medications are available
		Many use HFA propellants in the United States
Holding Chamber, Reverse-Flow Spacer, or Spacer	Reduces the need for patient coordination	Inhalation can be more complex for some patients
	Reduces pharyngeal deposition	Can reduce the dose available if not used properly
		More expensive than MDI alone
		Less portable than MDI alone
		Integrated actuator devices may alter aerosol properties compared to native actuator
DPI	Breath-actuated	Requires moderate to high inspiratory flow
	Less patient coordination required	Some units are single dose
	Propellant not required	Can result in high pharyngeal deposition
	Small and portable	Not all medications available
	Short treatment time	
	Dose counters in most newer designs	
SMI	Compact	Not breath actuated
	Small and Portable	Not currently available in many countries
	Multi-dose device	Not all medications are available
	Less coordination needed vs. pMDI	
	Short treatment time	
	High lung deposition	

Abbreviations: DPI = dry powder inhaler; pMDI = pressurized metered dose inhalers; SMI = soft mist inhaler; HFA = hydrofluoroalkane

Source: Modified from Dolovich et al. (81).

Although many patients in need of maintenance therapy for chronic lung disease can use pMDIs (with or without a spacer) or DPIs, certain patients will most likely benefit from administration by nebulizer (85, 86). These include:

- Patients with cognitive impairment, e.g., Alzheimer's dementia, intellectual disability, or altered consciousness, which preclude effective use of handheld inhalers.

- Patients with impaired manual dexterity due to arthritis, Parkinsonism, or stroke.

- Patients who have severe pain or muscle weakness due to neuromuscular disease.

- Patients who are unable to use pMDIs or DPIs in an optimal manner despite adequate instruction and training, such as those patients who are generally debilitated after hospitalization or by chronic illness and are unable to coordinate their breathing with a pMDI, or patients who cannot generate adequate inspiratory flow for effective aerosol delivery from a DPI.

- Patients with inadequate symptom relief with appropriate use of pMDIs/DPIs.

- Patients who do not comply with the use of pMDIs and DPIs or who prefer nebulizers.

- Patients who need respiratory medications that are not available in pMDI or DPI formulations; in the United States, for example, some antibiotics, mucolytics, and prostaglandins are not available in hand-held inhalers.

- Patients who are unable to afford therapy with pMDIs or DPIs.

Other Considerations

Other potential disadvantages of nebulizers are their relatively poor efficiency, high residual volume of 0.5–1.5 mL, and a significant amount of aerosol wasted during exhalation with continuous operation. Limited access to accessories, the use of damaged parts, and patients engaging in self-repairs, are other problems associated with nebulizer use (84). Another limitation of nebulizers, which has now been resolved, was the lack of availability of long-acting muscarinic antagonists (LAMAs) in solution. The approval of glycopyrrolate (Lonhala, Sunovion) in 2018 and revefenacin (Yupelri, Mylan/Theravance) in 2019 has overcome this limitation.

EVOLVING PERSPECTIVES ON MAINTENANCE TREATMENT WITH NEBULIZERS

Most patients with stable COPD are prescribed maintenance therapy via inhaler, due to the perceived convenience of inhalers compared with nebulizers. In fact, until recently, nebulizers were not generally recommended for maintenance therapy for COPD. For example, in the first (2001) annual report of the Global Initiative for Chronic Obstructive Lung Disease (GOLD), and all subsequent Reports until 2010, GOLD stated that "Nebulizers are not recommended for regular treatment because they are more expensive and require appropriate maintenance" (87). In 2010, GOLD no longer stated that nebulizers were inappropriate for patients with stable COPD, but recommendations for their use were still cautious. The evolution toward accepting nebulizers as a standard inhalation delivery device in patients with stable COPD continued, and caveats regarding such use were removed from the GOLD Reports in 2017 (87).

For many years, inhalers and nebulizers were considered to be equally effective when used optimally, and it was considered that most patients could be trained to use their inhalers appropriately. However, the scientific evidence underlying this assumption is weak (88). Moreover, recent investigations, especially those that include patient perceptions as an outcome measure, suggest that nebulizers may provide more satisfactory symptom relief for some users (Table 8.5). These results are not surprising given the potential for suboptimal inhaler use by patients. Indeed, poor inhaler technique compromises symptom relief in up to 94% of patients with COPD (86). Inhaler use training could reduce such errors, yet even extensive training may not mitigate patients' misuse of inhalers. For example, in the survey conducted by Hanania et al. (89), 79% of patients with COPD reported at least one physical or cognitive impairment that

Table 8.5: Surveys of patient-reported symptom control, quality of life, and device preference with nebulizers vs. inhalers

First Author, Year	Study Type	Sample Size	Study Findings
Barta, 2002 (90)	Patient survey (via postal questionnaire)	82 with COPD	Nebulized treatment at home helped patients feel comfortable and more in charge of their own symptom control; compliance was generally excellent
Sharafkhaneh, 2013 (91)	Telephone survey of randomly selected patients and caregivers	400 patients with COPD and 400 caregivers	Most patients and caregivers (~80%) preferred therapy with nebulizers vs. inhalers for controlling symptoms and improving quality of life
Dhand, 2018 (92)	Online survey using the Harris Poll Online panel	254 patients with COPD	54% of patients with COPD preferred nebulizers to other inhalation devices
Hanania, 2018 (89)	Web-based, descriptive, cross-sectional US-based survey	499 with self-reported COPD	Most (35%) patients reported no device preference, whereas 33% preferred pMDIs, 12% preferred nebulizers, 10% preferred SMIs, and 9% preferred DPIs. Patients with more severe symptoms (mMRC score ≥ 2) were most likely to report using a nebulizer.

Abbreviations: COPD = chronic obstructive pulmonary disease; DPI = dry powder inhaler; pMDIs = pressurized metered dose inhalers.

Source: From Terry and Dhand (88).

could limit their ability to correctly manipulate an inhaler device, including arthritis, poor eyesight, poor hearing, memory problems, tremor, difficulty with fine motor activities, depression, or anxiety, and more than half of the respondents had multiple limitations. Consequently, even assuming inhaler-nebulizer equivalence with perfect use, most patients with COPD may not achieve optimal benefits from inhalers due to co-morbid physical and cognitive limitations that cannot be improved by device training alone.

In summary, nebulizers remain a cornerstone of respiratory drug delivery. Compared with pMDIs or DPIs, nebulizers are more forgiving of faulty technique, can deliver larger doses and a wider range of medications and formulations, and appear to provide greater symptomatic benefit in studies of patient-reported outcomes. The use of nebulizers in the ambulatory setting has been facilitated by modern technologies and designs that have increased their portability and reduced their noise, size, and treatment times. Nonetheless, nebulizers still vary in terms of design and interface, cost, nebulization and delivery efficiency, output rate, drug degradation, "smart" or "intelligent" design features, and overall performance. Consideration of these factors is needed to optimize nebulizer use based on the patient's individual needs and preferences.

REFERENCES

1. American Association for Respiratory Care: Virtual Museum: Aerosol delivery devices. [cited 2022 Feb 23] https://museum.aarc.org/galleries/aerosol-delivery-devices/
2. Anderson PJ. History of aerosol therapy: Liquid nebulization to MDIs to DPIs. Respir Care 2005;50:1139–1150.
3. Burks AW. Aerosols and aerosol drug delivery systems. In: Burks AW, Holgate ST, O'Hehir R, et al. editors. Middleton's allergy: Principles and practice. Amsterdam: Elsevier; 2020.
4. Hess D, Fisher D, Williams P, et al. Medication nebulizer performance. Effects of diluent volume, nebulizer flow, and nebulizer brand. Chest 1996;110:498–505.
5. Hess DR, Acosta FL, Ritz RH, et al. The effect of heliox on nebulizer function using a beta-agonist bronchodilator. Chest 1999;115:184–189.
6. Phipps PR, Gonda I. Droplets produced by medical nebulizers. Some factors affecting their size and solute concentration. Chest 1990;97:1327–1332.
7. Stapleton KW, Finlay WH. Determining solution concentration within aerosol droplets output by jet nebulizers. J Aerosol Sci 1995;26:137–145.
8. Broaddus VC. Aerosols and drug delivery. In: Broaddus VC, Ernst J, King TE Jr, et al. editors. Murray & Nadel's textbook of respiratory medicine. Vol 1, 7th ed. Amsterdam: Elsevier; 2022.
9. Rau JL. Design principles of liquid nebulization devices currently in use. Respir Care 2002;47:1257–1275; discussion 1275–1278.
10. Alvine GF, Rogers P, Fitzsimmons KM, et al. Disposable jet nebulizers. How reliable are they? Chest 1992;101:316–319.
11. Waldrep JC, Keyhani K, Black M, et al. Operating characteristics of 18 different continuous-flow jet nebulizers with beclomethasone dipropionate liposome aerosol. Chest 1994;105:106–110.
12. Ari A. Jet, ultrasonic, and mesh nebulizers: An evaluation of nebulizers for better clinical outcomes. Eurasian J Pulmonol 2014;16:1–7.
13. McCallion ONM, Taylor KMG, Thomas M, et al. Nebulization of fluids of different physicochemical properties with air-jet and ultrasonic nebulizers. Pharm Res 1995;12:1682–1688.

14. McCallion ONM, Taylor KMG, Thomas M, et al. The influence of surface tension on aerosols produced by medical nebulisers. Int J Pharm 1996;129:123–136.
15. MacNeish CF, Meisner D, Thibert R, et al. A comparison of pulmonary availability between Ventolin (albuterol) nebules and Ventolin (albuterol) Respirator Solution. Chest 1997;111:204–208. DOI:10.1378/chest.111.1.204
16. Ferron GA, Gebhart J. Estimation of the lung deposition of aerosol particles produced with medical nebulizers. J Aerosol Sci 1988;19:1083–1086.
17. Devadason SG, Everard M, Linto JM, et al. Comparison of drug delivery from conventional versus "Venturi" nebulizers. Eur Respir J 1997;10(11):2479–2483.
18. Ho SL, Kwong WT, O'Drowsky L, et al. Evaluation of four breath-enhanced nebulizers for home use. J Aerosol Med 2001;14(4):467–475.
19. Leung K, Louca E, Coates AL. Comparison of breath-enhanced to breath-actuated nebulizers for rate, consistency, and efficiency. Chest 2004;126(5):1619–1627.
20. Rau JL, Arzu A, Restrepo RD. Performance comparison of nebulizer designs: Constant output, breath-enhanced, and dosimetric. Respir Care 2004;49:174–179.
21. Dessanges JF. A history of nebulization. J Aerosol Med 2001;14:65–71.
22. Mercer TT. Production of therapeutic aerosols: Principles and techniques. Chest 1981;80:813–818.
23. Lentz YK, Anchordoquy TJ, Langsfeld CS. Rationale for the selection of an aerosol delivery system for gene delivery. J Aerosol Med 2006;19:372–384.
24. Harvey CJ, O'Doherty MJ, Page CJ, et al. Comparison of jet and ultrasonic nebulizer pulmonary aerosol deposition during mechanical ventilation. Eur Respir J 1997;10:905–909.
25. Mercer TT, Tillery MI, Chow HY. Operating characteristics of some compressed-air nebulizers. Am Ind Hyg Assoc J 1968;29:66–78.
26. Niven RW, Ip AY, Mittelman S, et al. Some factors associated with the ultrasonic nebulization of proteins. Pharm Res 1995;12:53–59.
27. Steckel H, Eskandar F. Factors affecting aerosol performance during nebulization with jet and ultrasonic nebulizers. Eur J Pharm Sci 2003;19:443–455.
28. Nikander K, Turpeinen M, Wollmer P. The conventional ultrasonic nebulizer proved inefficient in nebulizing a suspension. J Aerosol Med 1999;12:47–53.
29. Leung KKM, Bridges PA, Taylor KMG. The stability of liposomes to ultrasonic nebulization. Int J Pharm 1996;145:95–102.
30. Vecellio L. The mesh nebuliser: A recent technical innovation for aerosol delivery. Breathe 2006;2:252–260.
31. Pritchard JN, Hatley RHM, Denyer J, et al. Mesh nebulizers have become the first choice for new nebulized pharmaceutical drug developments. Ther Deliv 2018;9:121–136.
32. Dhand R. Nebulizers that use a vibrating mesh or plate with multiple apertures to generate aerosol. Respir Care 2002;47:1406–1416.
33. Nickerson C, Von Hollen D, Garbin S, et al. Preference and quality of life of adult chronic obstructive lung disease (COPD) patients when using a novel mesh nebulizer compared to traditional jet nebulizer (TJN). Eur Respir J 2020;56:640. DOI:10.1183/13993003.congress-2020.640
34. Dhand R. How should aerosols be delivered during invasive mechanical ventilation. Respir Care 2017;62:1343–1367.

35. Denyer J, Dyche T. The adaptive aerosol delivery (AAD) technology: Past, present, and future. J Aerosol Med Pulm Drug Deliv 2010;23(Suppl 1):S1–S10.

36. Brand P, Beckmann H, Maas-Enriquez M, et al. Peripheral deposition of alpha1-protease inhibitor using commercial inhalation devices. Eur Respir J 2003;22:263–267.

37. Griese M, Ramakers J, Krasselt A, et al. Improvement of alveolar glutathione and lung function but not oxidative state in cystic fibrosis. Am J Respir Crit Care Med 2004;169:822–828.

38. Ruffin RE, Dolovich MB, Wolff RK, et al. The effects of preferential deposition of histamine in the human airway. Am Rev Respir Dis 1978;117(3):485–492.

39. van den Bosch WB, Kloosterman SF, Andrinopoulou ER, et al. Small airways targeted treatment with smart nebulizer technology could improve severe asthma in children: A retrospective analysis. J Asthma 2022;59:2223–2233. DOI:10.1080/02770903.2021.1996597

40. Smith DW, Frankel LR, Mathers LH, et al. A controlled trial of aerosolized ribavarin in infants receiving mechanical ventilation for severe respiratory syncytial virus infection. N Engl J Med 1991;325:24–29.

41. Coates AL, MacNeish CF, Meisner D, et al. The choice of jet nebulizer, nebulizing flow, and addition of albuterol affects the output of tobramycin aerosols. Chest 1997;111(5):1206–1212.

42. Berlinski A, Waldrep JC. Nebulized drug admixtures: Effect on aerosol characteristics and albuterol output. J Aerosol Med 2006;19(4):484–490.

43. Burchett DK, Darko W, Zahra J, et al. Mixing and compatibility guide for commonly used aerosolized medications. Am J Health Syst Pharm 2010;67(3):227–230. DOI:10.2146/ajhp080261

44. McKenzie JE, Cruz-Rivera M. Compatibility of budesonide inhalation suspension with four nebulizing solutions. Ann Pharmacother 2004;38(6):967–972.

45. Akapo S, Gupta J, Martinez E, et al. Compatibility and aerosol characteristics of formoterol fumarate mixed with other nebulizing solutions. Ann Pharmacother 2008;42:1416–1424.

46. Kamin W, Erdnüss F, Krämer I. Inhalation solutions–which ones may be mixed? Physico-chemical compatibility of drug solutions in nebulizers–update 2013. J Cyst Fibros 2014;13(3):243–250. DOI:10.1016/j.jcf.2013.09.006

47. Everard ML, Hardy JG, Milner AD. Comparison of nebulized aerosol deposition in the lungs of healthy adults following oral and nasal inhalation. Thorax 1993;48(10):1045–1046.

48. Chua HL, Collis GG, Newbury AM, et al. The influence of age on aerosol deposition in children with cystic fibrosis. Eur Respir J 1994;7:2185–2191.

49. Nikander K, Agertoft L, Pedersen S. Breath-synchronized nebulization diminishes the impact of patient-device interfaces (face mask or mouthpiece) on the inhaled mass of nebulized budesonide. J Asthma 2000;37(5):451–459.

50. Kishida M, Suzuki I, Kabayama H, et al. Mouthpiece versus face mask for delivery of nebulized salbutamol in exacerbated childhood asthma. J Asthma 2002;39(4):337–339.

51. Sangwan S, Gurses BK, Smaldone GC. Face masks and facial deposition of aerosols. Pediatr Pulmonol 2004;37(5):447–452.

52. Hayden JT, Smith N, Woolf DA, et al. A randomised crossover trial of face mask efficacy. Arch Dis Child 2004;89(1):72–73.

53. Erzinger S, Schueepp KG, Brooks-Wildhaber J, et al. Face masks and aerosol delivery in vivo. J Aerosol Med 2007;20(Suppl 1):S78–S84.
54. Bisquerra RA, Botz GH, Nates JL. Ipratropium-bromide-induced acute anisocoria in the intensive care setting due to ill-fitting face masks. Respir Care 2005;50(12):1662–1664.
55. Smaldone GC, Sangwan S, Shah A. Face mask design, facial deposition, and delivered dose of nebulized aerosols. J Aerosol Med 2007;20(Suppl 1):S66–S77.
56. Smaldone GC. Advances in aerosols: Adult respiratory disease. J Aerosol Med 2006;19:36–46.
57. Peters SG. Continuous bronchodilator therapy. Chest 2007;131(1):286–289.
58. Berlinski A, Waldrep JC. Four hours of continuous albuterol nebulization. Chest 1998;114(3):847–853.
59. Raabe OG, Wong TM, Wong GB, et al. Continuous nebulization therapy for asthma with aerosols of beta2 agonists. Ann Allergy Asthma Immunol 1998;80(6):499–508.
60. Kelly HW, Keim KA, McWilliams BC. Comparison of two methods of delivering continuously nebulized albuterol. Ann Pharmacother 2003;37(1):23–26.
61. Camargo CA Jr, Spooner CH, Rowe BH. Continuous versus intermittent beta-agonists in the treatment of acute asthma. Cochrane Database Syst Rev 2003;(4):CD001115.
62. Lavorini F, Usmani OS, Dhand R. Aerosol delivery systems for treating obstructive airway diseases during the SARS-CoV-2 pandemic. Intern Emerg Med 2021;16:2035–2039.
63. Halpin DMG, Criner GJ, Papi A, et al. The 2020 GOLD science committee report on COVID-19 and chronic obstructive pulmonary disease. Am J Respir Crit Care Med 2021;203(1):24–36.
64. Respiratory Care Committee of Chinese Thoracic Society. Expert consensus on preventing nosocomial transmission during respiratory care for critically ill patients infected by 2019 novel coronavirus pneumonia. Zhonghua Jie He Hu Xi Za Zhi 2020;43(4):288–296.
65. Jain GK, Chandra L, Dhand R. Clinical evaluation of dispersion and disposition of exhaled droplets during nebulization using 3-D gamma scintigraphy. Paper presented at NAPCON 2020 (virtual). 22nd Joint National Conference of National College of Chest Physicians (India) and Indian Chest Society. January 27–31, 2021. New Delhi, India.
66. Fink JB, Ehrmann S, Li J, et al. Reducing aerosol-related risk of transmission in the era of COVID-19: An interim guidance endorsed by the International Society of Aerosols in Medicine. J Aerosol Med Pulm Drug Deliv 2020;33(6):300–304. DOI:10.1089/jamp.2020.1615
67. Hui DS, Chan MT, Chow B. Aerosol dispersion during various respiratory therapies: A risk assessment model of nosocomial infection to health care workers. Hong Kong Med J 2014;20(Suppl 4):9–13.
68. National Institute for Health and Care Excellence, COVID-19 rapid guideline: Severe asthma (NICE guideline [NG166]). 2020. Available from: https://www.nice.org.uk/guidance/ng166
69. CDC. Interim US Guidance for risk assessment and public health management of healthcare personnel with potential exposure in a healthcare setting to patients with coronavirus disease 2019 (COVID-19). [cited 2020 Apr 15]. Available from: https://www.cdc.gov/coronavirus/2019-ncov/hcp/guidance-risk-assessment-hcp.html

70. McGrath JA, O'Toole C, Bennett G, et al. Investigation of fugitive aerosols released into the environment during high-flow therapy. Pharmaceutics 2019;11:254.

71. Avari H, Hiebert RJ, Ryzynski AA, et al. Quantitative assessment of viral dispersion associated with respiratory support devices in a simulated critical care environment. Am J Respir Crit Care Med 2021;203:1112–1118.

72. Harnois LJ, Alolaiwat AA, Jing G, et al. Efficacy of various mitigation devices in reducing fugitive emissions from nebulizers. Respir Care 2022;67(4):394–403.

73. McGrath JA, O'Sullivan A, Bennett G, et al. Investigation of the quantity of exhaled aerosols released into the environment during nebulisation. Pharmaceutics 2019;11(2):75.

74. Wittgen BP, Kunst PW, Perkins WR, et al. Assessing a system to capture stray aerosol during inhalation of nebulized liposomal cisplatin. J Aerosol Med 2006;19:385–391.

75. Schuschnig U, Ledermuller R, Gramann J. Efficacy of the PARI filter-valve set to prevent environmental contamination with aerosol during nebulizer therapy. 2020. Preprint. https://www.researchgate.net/publication/342987954

76. Liu M, Cheng S-Z, Xu K-W, et al. Use of personal protective equipment against coronavirus disease 2019 by healthcare professionals in Wuhan, China: Cross sectional study. BMJ 2020;369:m2195. DOI:10.1136/bmj.m2195

77. Smith EC, Denyer J, Kendrick AH. Comparison of twenty three nebulizer/compressor combinations for domiciliary use. Eur Respir J 1995;8:1214.

78. Malone RA, Hollie MC, Glynn-Barnhart A, et al. Optimal duration of nebulized albuterol therapy. Chest 1993;104:1114–1118.

79. Rau JL, Restrepo RD. Nebulized bronchodilator formulations: Unit-dose or multi-dose? Respir Care 2003;48:926–939.

80. Bell J, Alexander L, Carson J, et al. Nebuliser hygiene in cystic fibrosis: Evidence-based recommendations. Breathe (Sheff) 2020;16:190328. DOI:10.1183/20734735.0328-2019

81. Dolovich MB, Ahrens RC, Hess DR, et al. Device selection and outcomes of aerosol therapy: Evidence-based guidelines: American College of Chest Physicians/American College of Asthma, Allergy, and Immunology. Chest 2005;127:335–371.

82. Melani AS, Bonavia M, Cilenti V, et al. Inhaler mishandling remains common in real life and is associated with reduced disease control. Respir Med 2011;105:930–938.

83. Duarte AG, Tung L, Zhang W, et al. Spirometry measurement of peak inspiratory flow identifies suboptimal use of dry powder inhalers in ambulatory patients with COPD. Chronic Obstr Pulm Dis 2019;6:246–255.

84. Alhaddad B, Smith FJ, Robertson T, et al. Patients' practices and experiences of using nebuliser therapy in the management of COPD at home. BMJ Open Respir Res 2015;2:e000076. DOI:10.1136/bmjresp-2014-000076

85. Dhand R, Dolovich M, Chipps B, et al. The role of nebulized therapy in the management of COPD: Evidence and recommendations. COPD 2012;9:58–72.

86. Usmani OS. Choosing the right inhaler for your asthma or COPD patient. Ther Clin Risk Manag 2019;15:461–472.

87. Terry P, Dhand R. Inhalation therapy for stable COPD: 20 years of GOLD reports. Adv Ther 2020;37:1812–1828.

88. Terry P, Dhand R. Maintenance therapy with nebulizers in patients with stable COPD: Need for reevaluation. Pulm Ther 2020;6:177–192.

89. Hanania NA, Braman S, Adams SG, et al. The role of inhalation delivery devices in COPD: Perspectives of patients and health care providers. Chronic Obstr Pulm Dis 2018;5:111–123.

90. Barta SK, Crawford A, Roberts CM. Survey of patients' views of domiciliary nebuliser treatment for chronic lung disease. Respir Med 2002;96:375–381.

91. Sharafkhaneh A, Wolf RA, Goodnight S, et al. Perceptions and attitudes toward the use of nebulized therapy for COPD: Patient and caregiver perspectives. COPD 2013;10:482–492.

92. Dhand R, Mahler DA, Carlin BW, et al. Results of a patient survey regarding COPD knowledge, treatment experiences, and practices with inhalation devices. Respir Care 2018;63:833–839.

9 Inhalation Therapy in Infants and Children

Bruce K. Rubin and Israel Amirav

CONTENTS

INTRODUCTION

In this chapter, we first describe why infants/small children are different with respect to their anatomy/physiology and their behavior. We will then review the available aerosol-generating devices and conclude with suggestions to improve clinical outcomes of aerosol therapy in this age group.

Anatomy/Physiology/Behavior

Infants and children younger than three years of age present unique challenges to aerosol delivery. Small children have anatomical limitations, as well as emotional challenges, and barriers to compliance. The devices used for aerosol delivery in infants and younger children were originally designed for adults. Less is known about the anatomic, physiological, and behavioral issues related to use of aerosol devices that are specific to infants. For example, if a baby is fighting the nebulizer face mask and crying, parents might substitute "blow by" treatment in which the mask is removed from the nebulizer tubes and the open end of the tube is held close to the infant's face, a technique that is no longer recommended because of its very low efficiency in delivering aerosol to the lungs (1). Alternatively, parents might tighten the grip on the mask, thinking that this will result in improved delivery. If the therapy fails, this may lead physicians to falsely assume that an increased drug dosage is required.

In terms of their anatomy, infants have a pharynx that is much higher in the upper respiratory tract, near the base of the tongue (Figure 9.1). They are largely nose breathers, and their larynx and supraglottic region are less rigid, and subsequently more susceptible to obstruction or collapse, particularly on inspiration. The epiglottis, which is relatively narrow and floppy, is located nearer the palate. This may explain why infants preferentially breathe through their nose (2).

Nose breathing serves as a barrier to aerosol delivery since the nose and nasopharynx have high resistance to flow. It has been shown that infants' noses are efficient in filtering air, which decreases the inhalation of toxins, as well as inhaled therapies (3). Infants also have faster growth of lung parenchyma relative to airway growth, which leads to increased airway conductance (4). The implications of this remain largely unexplored, but a greater proportion of aerosol particles may reach the lung parenchyma because they travel a shorter distance. Because of their diameter, infants' lungs are more susceptible to obstruction of airways with airway disease. Another consideration is airflow.

DOI: 10.1201/9781003269014-9

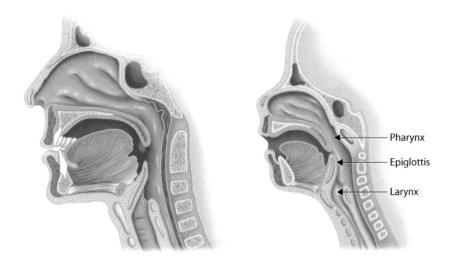

Figure 9.1 The upper airway of adults (left) compared with that of infants (right): pharynx and supraglottic region: Less rigid; epiglottis: Narrow, floppy, and closer to palate; larynx: Higher and very close to the base of the tongue.

Infants have a faster inspiratory airflow but with lower volumes than older children, leading to aerosol delivery to the more proximal airways upon inhalation.

Infants breathe more rapidly and with a smaller tidal volume, decreasing lung deposition. This breathing pattern, compounded with nose breathing, results in more aerosol particles getting trapped in the upper respiratory tract. We have recently compared nasal and oral delivery of aerosol in anatomically correct replicas of infants' faces containing both nasal and oral upper airways (5). Three CT-derived upper respiratory tract replicas representing infants/toddlers aged 5, 14, and 20 months were studied and aerosol delivery (using a lung mechanical simulator) to the "lower respiratory tract" (LRT) by either the oral or nasal route for each of the replicas was measured at the "tracheal" opening. Nasal delivery to the LRT exceeded oral delivery in the 5- and 14-month models and was equivalent in the 20-month model. Differences between nasal and oral delivery diminished with age/size and were unrelated to tidal volumes (5).

In vivo studies employing aerosolized radiolabeled particles to measure lung deposition in infants with various pulmonary diseases are few, but the results are strikingly similar regardless of disease state (Table 9.1).

These *in vivo* studies have demonstrated that lung deposition of radiolabeled aerosols is no more than 2% for age 12 months and under, but by the age of about 3 years, it has increased to about 5%. Compared to children over age 8 and adults who may deposit 20–40% of the mouth dose below the larynx, these deposition values appear to be minute. However, since the infant's airway surface area is relatively small, it turns out that these "adult doses," although markedly attenuated, provide a similar clinical response without increased adverse effects.

Children generally do not know how to adequately inhale through a mouthpiece until about 3–4 years of age. Because of this, a face mask that is

Table 9.1: Lung Deposition of Aerosol Therapeutics Given to Infants and Young Children with Different Diseases/Disorders

Author	Disease	Age (Mean, m)	n	Lung Deposition (%)
Chua (6)	CF	9	12	**1.3**
Mallol (7)	CF	12	5	**2**
Tal (8)	Asthma, CF, BPD	21	15	**2**
Fok (9)	BPD	3	13	**1.7**
Amirav (10)	Bronchiolitis	8	12	**1.5**
Amirav (11)	Asthma	6	12	**1.7**
Amirav (12)	Healthy	9	10	**1.6**

Abbreviations: BPD = bronchopulmonary dysplasia; CF = cystic fibrosis.
Note: Bold values are outcome of interest.

comfortable and has a tight seal may improve aerosol delivery (13). Even a 1-cm gap between the mask and the face led to a 50% reduction in aerosol delivery with a small-volume nebulizer (14). A tight-fitting seal is most important when it comes to aerosol delivery through pressurized metered dose inhalers (pMDIs) with valved holding chambers (VHCs) because drug delivery occurs only when the infant or child inhales through the device. With jet nebulizers, a poor seal results in the escape of drug and admixture with outside air, and with the new breath-actuated nebulizers, a tight seal is required for drug delivery. Unfortunately, current facemask designs do not consider the distinct anatomical and physiological needs of infants and young children. A study involving the NebuChamber mask demonstrated a 30% higher efficiency of airway delivery with an improved design and a tighter seal (15). It is important to note that in both this study and another (16), it was shown that dose variability increased with decreased cooperation by the children. This suggests that a tight-fitting mask design is a less important factor than child compliance.

Crying during aerosol delivery is a complex issue. Crying is characterized by a long exhalation, followed by a short inspiratory gasp. This increases the chances that the drug will remain in the upper respiratory tract, since the drug is only available during the short inhalation phase, and not during exhalation. Additionally, crying is accompanied by agitation, which makes a poor mask seal more likely. Infants cry in reaction to being "smothered" by an uncomfortable facemask, and the caregiver may then create a tighter, more forceful seal, exacerbating the discomfort. This leads to struggling, and a further compromised seal. Crying has been shown to be a primary cause of poor face-to-mask seal, and while crying is a common occurrence during aerosol delivery, it is not inevitable. It has been suggested that allowing children to play with the facemask before delivery makes the child less likely to cry. Parents should be coached on techniques to relax the child and ease them into the therapy. Such techniques include having the child hold the facemask up to their parents or favorite stuffed animal or rewarding the child for proper use of the device.

There are studies that demonstrate a clear positive correlation between the level of infant distress and deposition of aerosol in the upper respiratory tract, which leads to swallowing and gastrointestinal tract deposition and absorption (17).

AEROSOL-GENERATING DEVICES

Pneumatic or Small Volume Jet Nebulizers (SVNs)

Jet nebulizers are sometimes used for children because of the misconception that children are unable to effectively use a pMDI even with a VHC (18). Although the response to medications given by a pMDI with holding chamber can be similar to that achieved by a nebulizer, because the use of the pMDI is much faster, more portable, less expensive than individually administered nebulizer doses, does not require cleaning, there is less pharyngeal deposition and less swallowed drug, and greater adherence with therapy when using a pMDI and chamber, a jet nebulizer should be used when the medication is only available as a nebulizer solution (e.g. dornase alfa, hypertonic saline).

Large-Volume Nebulizer

The large-volume pneumatic nebulizer (LVN) has a reservoir volume greater than 100 mL and can be used to administer a solution over a prolonged period. LVNs work on the same principles as small-volume nebulizers, with the exception that the residual volume is greater and the effects of evaporation over time are more profound. When using the LVN to administer a solution containing medications, such as bronchodilators, the medication becomes increasingly concentrated over time because of preferential evaporation of the diluent (19).

Ultrasonic Nebulizers (USN)

USN produce ultrasonic waves directly into the solution, which produces aerosol on the surface of the liquid. USNs are capable of higher aerosol outputs (0.5–7 mL/minute) and higher aerosol densities than most conventional jet nebulizers. Particle size is affected by the frequency of the waves, while output is affected by the amplitude of the signal. Frequency is usually device-specific and is not user-adjustable. Unlike jet nebulizers, the temperature of the solution placed in a USN increases during use. As the temperature increases, the drug concentration may also rise, increasing the likelihood of undesired side effects. In addition, some drugs may be adversely affected by the increased operating temperature (20). Pulmonary deposition of drugs delivered by currently available ultrasonic nebulizers is so poor that these cannot be recommended for the administration of asthma medications (21).

Several other hazards are associated with using an USN. Over hydration may occur when using a USN for prolonged treatment of a neonate, small child, or other patient with fluid and electrolyte imbalances. The high-density aerosols from USNs have been associated with bronchospasm, increased airway resistance, and irritability in a substantial proportion of the population (22).

Vibrating Mesh Nebulizers (VMN)

A relatively recent advance in nebulizer therapy is the vibrating mesh nebulizer (VMN). In this device, a piezo element vibrates a mesh or horn in contact with drug. As the liquid passes through multiple holes in the mesh, the vibrating action generates medicated aerosol. Because the mesh is uniform by design, this can be tailored to specific medications and the resulting aerosol usually has a smaller and more uniform particle size (mass median aerodynamic diameter; MMAD and geometric standard deviation; GSD) than jet nebulizers. The VMN devices are small, more portable than pneumatic jet nebulizers, generally battery or AC powered, and are silent and fast. There is also the ability to give a higher dose of drug to the patient. Because of these properties, the VMN is an attractive alternative delivery device for children (23).

However, VMN devices are more expensive to purchase, cannot be effectively used with very viscous drugs or drug suspensions, drug-carrier complexes (e.g. liposomes) may be disrupted, and pores in the mesh can be clogged, for example if a patient chooses to administer hyperosmolar saline through their VMN. The mesh is difficult to clear and can also be clogged with soap residue.

Pressurized Metered Dose Inhalers (pMDIs)

The pMDI is the most commonly prescribed method of aerosol delivery. More formulations of aerosol drugs are currently available for use by pMDI than for use with other aerosol delivery systems. Properly used, pMDIs are at least as effective as nebulizers for drug delivery (24). For this reason, pMDIs are often the preferred method for delivering bronchodilators to both spontaneously breathing and intubated patients.

pMDI actuation into a VHC decreases impaction losses by reducing the velocity of the aerosol plume and allowing time for evaporation of the propellants before impacting on a surface. The dose of medication with the pMDI is much smaller than with the nebulizer.

Effective use of the pMDI is technique dependent (25). Common hand-breath coordination problems include actuating the pMDI before or after the breath. Some patients, especially infants, young children, the elderly, and patients in acute distress may not be able to use a pMDI. These problems reduce aerosol delivery to the lung but can be corrected by using a VHC (*vide infra*). Good patient instruction should include demonstration, practice, and confirmation of patient performance. Repeated instruction improves performance; but should occur several times.

Spacers and Valved Holding Chambers

Spacers and VHCs are accessory devices, that when used properly can decrease oropharyngeal deposition of drug and improve hand-breath coordination. A spacer device is an open-ended straight tube or bag that provides space for the pMDI plume to expand and slow, and soluble particles become smaller before entering the airway. A VHC incorporates a one-way valve that permits the aerosol to be drawn from the chamber during inhalation, diverting the exhaled gas to the atmosphere, not disturbing any remaining aerosol suspended in the chamber. Patients with small tidal volumes can generally empty the aerosol from the chamber with 3–6 successive breaths. For use with infants, VHCs should have minimal dead space, and a valve that will open or close with the pressures and flow generated by the patient (26).

The use of a VHC should be encouraged at all ages and especially for young children. These accessory devices can reduce the need to coordinate the breath with actuation, reduce oral deposition, increase respirable particles, and improve lower respiratory tract deposition. These devices lead to a 10- to 15-fold reduction in the pharyngeal dose of aerosol from the pMDI (26, 27).

The belief that a nebulizer is better than a pMDI if the patient is not able to inhale with optimal technique using the inspiratory hold is not supported by research. In fact, if the patient cannot perform an optimal maneuver using a pMDI, they will be unable to perform an effective inhalation using a nebulizer. Although optimal technique is always preferred, it is often difficult to attain with an infant, small child, or severely dyspneic patient. In such cases, the alternative to optimal deposition may be to increase the pMDI or nebulizer dosage.

Respimat[R] Soft Mist Inhaler (SMI)

The SMI was developed over 20 years ago but has been in commercial use for only the past decade, primarily to deliver tiotropium. The device is uniquely powered by spring compression, thus requiring no electricity to operate. The SMI produces an aerosol over 1.2 seconds at a velocity of about 10 M/s; much less that a pMDI and hence the name "soft mist." The slower aerosol velocity improves coordination, and the SMI is generally easier to use than the pMDI used without a VHC. Drug delivery to the lung of adults is highly efficient; in the range of 40%. However, actuation and inhalation still need to be coordinated and this can be a problem for young children (28). Coordination with a SMI could be improved with the use of a holding chamber in children (29). As well, the medication dose chamber in a SMI is relatively small at 11–14 µL, limiting the amount of medication that can be administered with each inhalation.

Dry Powder Inhalers

DPIs are alternatives to pMDIs in older children and adults. Because of portability and rapid ease of use, many patients prefer a DPI. Dose adjustment may be needed when the same drug is administered by a DPI instead of by pMDI and many medications are not available as a DPI. The internal geometry of the DPI device influences the resistance offered to inspiration and the inspiratory flow required to produce an aerosol (30). Because DPIs are mostly dependent on inspiratory pressure drop to generate the aerosol (31), very young children (<6 years old) cannot use DPIs effectively. Breath coordination is also an issue with DPIs. Exhalation into a DPI blows out the powder from the device and reduces drug delivery. Moreover, the humidity in the exhaled air may influence subsequent aerosol generation from the DPI, especially when a very cold device interacts with a warm breath.

DPIs are breath-actuated, and they reduce the problem of coordinating inspiration with actuation that complicates the use of pMDIs. The technique of using DPIs differs in important respects from the technique employed to inhale drugs from a pMDI. Although DPIs are easier to use than pMDIs, up to 25% of patients may use DPIs improperly (32).

NEW STRATEGIES AND DELIVERY DESIGNS

One novel delivery method involves using a hood, which reduces infant crying during therapy. Since this method does not involve placing a mask over the child's face, infants are often more compliant, with a similar clinical benefit and lung deposition. There is a renewed interest in the use of similar hoods as those originally described by us (17) during the Covid-19 pandemic, though the purpose of using the hoods was more to protect caregivers during aerosol therapy rather than to facilitate treatment of patients (33).

Another advance in the field is the development of the SootherMask, which is a face mask that attaches to the VHC (34). It is a soft and flexible mask that has a slot for the child's pacifier. The mask accepts most pacifiers and provides rapid and efficient delivery of pMDI aerosol treatment to children during normal breathing while they suck on the pacifier. It was developed based on anthropometric analysis of the infant's facial structure, and thus, is better aligned to the infant's face, achieves a seal with minimal force, and minimizes dead space.

FINAL RECOMMENDATIONS FOR DEVICE SELECTION

The administered dose of aerosolized medication should be the same for all ages. Although more drug deposits in the airway of adults and older children because there is a greater airway surface, there is no age-associated dose adjustment needed independent of the delivery system. Whenever possible, patients should employ only one type of aerosol-generating device for inhalation therapy. The technique of using each device is different, and repeated instruction is necessary to ensure that the patient uses the device appropriately. The use of several devices for inhalation can be confusing for patients and may decrease their adherence to therapy.

Sadly, many clinicians, including physicians, nurses, and pharmacists do not know the correct technique for using pMDIs or DPIs and thus cannot teach this to their patients. Often it is the respiratory therapist or certified asthma educator who is the best educator (35).

REFERENCES

1. Rubin B. Bye-bye, blow by. Respir Care 2007;52(8):981.
2. Becquemin MH, Swift DL, Bouchikhi A, et al. Particle deposition and resistance in the noses of adults and children. Eur Respir J 1991;4:694–702.
3. Schwab JA, Zenkel M. Filtration of particulates in the human nose. Laryngoscope 1998;108:120–124.
4. Stocks J, Godfrey S. Specific airway conductance in relation to postconceptional age during infancy. J Appl Physiol Respir Environ Exerc Physiol 1977;43(1):144–154. DOI:10.1152/jappl.1977.43.1.144
5. Amirav I, Borojeni A, Halamish A, et al. Nasal versus oral aerosol delivery to the "lungs" in infants and toddlers. Pediatr Pulmonol 2015;50:276–283.
6. Chua HL, Collis GG, Newbury AM, et al. The influence of age on aerosol deposition in children with cystic fibrosis. Eur Respir J 1994;7:2185–2191.
7. Mallol J, Rattray S, Walker G, et al. Aerosol deposition in infants with cystic fibrosis. Pediatr Pulmonol 1996;21:276–281.
8. Tal A, Golan H, Grauer N, et al. Deposition pattern of radiolabeled salbutamol inhaled from a metered-dose inhaler by means of a spacer with mask in young children with airway obstruction. J Pediatr 1996;128:479–484.
9. Fok TF, Monkman S, Dolovich M, et al. Efficiency of aerosol medication delivery from a metered dose inhaler versus jet nebulizer in infants with bronchopulmonary dysplasia. Pediatr Pulmonol 1996;21:301–309.
10. Amirav I, Balanov I, Gorenberg M, et al. Beta agonist aerosol distribution in RSV bronchiolitis in infants. J Nucl Med 2002;43:487–491.
11. Amirav I, Luder A, Chleechel A, et al. Lung aerosol deposition in suckling infants. Arch Dis Child 2012;97(6):497–501.
12. Amirav I, Newhouse M, Luder A, et al. Feasibility of aerosol drug delivery to sleeping infants: A prospective observational study. BMJ Open 2014;4(3):e004124. DOI:10.1136/bmjopen-2013-004124
13. Amirav I, Newhouse MT. Aerosol therapy with valved holding chambers in young children: Importance of facemask seal. Pediatrics 2001;108:389–394.
14. Everard ML, Clark AR, Milner AD. Drug delivery from holding chambers with attached facemask. Arch Dis Child 1992;67(5):580–585.
15. Amirav I, Mansour Y, Mandelberg A, et al. Redesigned face mask improves "real life" aerosol delivery for nebuchamber. Pediatr Pulmonol 2004;37(2):172–177.
16. Esposito-Festen JE, Ates B, Van Vliet FJ, et al. Effect of a facemask leak on aerosol delivery from a pMDI-spacer system. J Aerosol Med 2004;17(1):1–6.
17. Amirav I, Balanov I, Gorenberg M, et al. Nebulizer hood compared to mask in wheezy infants: Aerosol therapy without tears. Arch Dis Child 2003;88:719–723.

18. Newhouse MT, Dolovich MB. Aerosol therapy: Nebulizer vs metered dose inhaler. Chest 1987;91:799–800.
19. Berlinski A, Willis JR, Leisenring T. In-vitro comparison of 4 large-volume nebulizers in 8 hours of continuous nebulization. Respir Care 2010;55(12):1671–1679.
20. Fink JB, Dhand R. Aerosol therapy. In: Fink JB, Hunt G, editors. Clinical practice in respiratory care. Philadelphia (PA): Lippincott Raven; 1998.
21. Nakanishi AK, Lamb BM, Foster C, et al. Ultrasonic nebulization of albuterol is no more effective than jet nebulization for the treatment of acute asthma in children. Chest 1997;111(6):1505–1508. DOI:10.1378/chest.111.6.1505
22. Boucher RGM, Kreuter J. Fundamentals of the ultrasonic atomization of medicated solutions. Ann Allergy 1968;26:59.
23. Moody GB, Luckett PM, Shockley CM, et al. Clinical efficacy of vibrating mesh and jet nebulizers with different interfaces in pediatric subjects with asthma. Respir Care 2020;65(10):1451–1463. DOI:10.4187/respcare.07538
24. Rubin BK, Fink JB. Optimizing aerosol delivery by pressurized metered dose inhalers. Respir Care 2005;50:1191–1197.
25. Fink JB, Rubin BK. Problems with inhaler use: A call for improved clinician and patient education. Respir Care 2005;50:1360–1375.
26. Nikander K, Nicholls C, Denyer J, et al. The evolution of spacers and valved holding chambers. J Aerosol Med Pulm Drug Deliv 2014;27(S1):S1–S4.
27. Rubin BK, Fink JB. Treatment delivery systems. Chapter 34 In: Castro M, Kraft M, editors. Clinical asthma. Philadelphia, PA: Elsevier-Mosby; 2008. p. 303–312.
28. Kamin W, Frank M, Kattenbeck S, et al. A handling study to assess use of the Respimat® Soft Mist™ inhaler in children under 5 years old. J Aerosol Med Pulm Drug Deliv 2015;28(5):372–381. DOI:10.1089/jamp.2014.1159
29. Wachtel H, Nagel M, Engel M, et al. In vitro and clinical characterization of the valved holding chamber AeroChamber Plus ® Flow-Vu® for administrating tiotropium Respimat® in 1-5-year-old children with persistent asthmatic symptoms. Respir Med 2018;137:181–190. DOI:10.1016/j.rmed.2018.03.010
30. Bisgaard H, Ifversen M, Klug B, et al. Inspiratory flow rate through the Diskus/Accuhaler inhaler and Turbuhaler inhaler in children with asthma. J Aerosol Med 1995;8:100.
31. Clark AR, Weers JG, Dhand R. The confusing world of dry powder inhalers: It is all about inspiratory pressures, not inspiratory flow rates. J Aerosol Med Pulm Drug Deliv 2020;33(1):1–11. DOI:10.1089/jamp.2019.1556
32. Kesten S, Elias M, Cartier A, et al. Patient handling of a multidose dry powder inhalation device for albuterol. Chest 1994;105:1077–1081.
33. Shaw KM, Lang AL, Lozano R, et al. Intensive care unit isolation hood decreases risk of aerosolization during noninvasive ventilation with COVID-19. Can J Anesth 2020;67, 1481–1483. DOI:10.1007/s12630-020-01721-5
34. Amirav I, Luder AS, Halamish A, et al. Design of aerosol face masks for children using computerized 3D face analysis. J Aerosol Med Pulm Drug Deliv 2014;27(4):272–278.
35. Hanania NA, Wittman R, Kesten S, et al. Medical personnel's knowledge of and ability to use inhaling devices: Metered-dose inhalers, spacing chambers, and breath-actuated dry powder inhalers. Chest 1994;105:111–116.

10 Selection of Inhaler Delivery System for Adult Outpatients

David M. G. Halpin and P. N. Richard Dekhuijzen

CONTENTS

INTRODUCTION

Consideration of the delivery system is essential when prescribing inhaled therapy for asthma or COPD to adult outpatients. Often a number of inhaler devices containing drugs of the appropriate class are available for prescription, and while there is evidence of the efficacy of the device and the drugs it contains in a population of patients, there is no evidence of which therapies are best suited to individual patients. In these circumstances, prescribers must still decide which therapy and inhaler delivery system to recommend. National and international guidelines do not make recommendations on how to select the optimal inhaler for a patient despite emphasizing the importance of a patient being able to use their device correctly (1–3). In part, this is because much of the time there isn't a single "best" choice and all devices can produce similar outcomes in patients when using the correct technique for inhalation (4).

Selecting the delivery system is likely to be influenced by clinicians' knowledge and personal beliefs about the actual and perceived benefits and disadvantages of particular drug and inhaler combinations. It will also be influenced by whether the patient is already taking inhaled therapy and whether they can use their current device correctly. The final choice should be made jointly by the prescriber and the patient taking into account all of these factors and is likely to differ from one patient to the next. Taking account of patients' goals and preferences in this way has been shown to improve outcomes for patients with asthma and is likely also to do so for patients with COPD (5, 6).

Worldwide, there are currently at least 33 different inhaled therapies containing different bronchodilators (both short- and long-acting) and inhaled corticosteroids (ICS), alone or in combinations. In addition, at least 22 different inhaler devices are available (1, 7). In many cases, a range of drugs is available in each device; in other cases, only one drug is available in a particular device. For simplification, devices can be grouped into four main types: pressurized metered-dose inhalers (pMDI), slow mist inhalers (SMI), dry powder inhalers (DPI), and nebulizers; however, not all devices within a group have similar properties and these differences must be taken into account as part of the decision making process.

DOI: 10.1201/9781003269014-10

The multiple permutations of medications and delivery systems, as well as clinicans' and patients' preferences and beliefs make it challenging to follow a precision medicine approach and choose an appropriate medication in a delivery system that matches individual patient factors. In practice, it appears many clinicians do not address this challenge, with for example 89% of physicians reporting that medication class was more important than device type in one recent survey (8). Such attitudes undoubtedly contribute to the poor adherence and persistence with inhaled therapy that has been prevalent since inhalers were introduced in the 1960s (9).

In this chapter, we review the evidence that should inform the selection. We review the features of the different inhalers that may affect selection and patient factors that affect their ability to use specific inhalers correctly, as well as evidence about clinicians' and patients' beliefs that may influence the choice of device. We also review algorithms that have been proposed to help with the selection of a device for an individual patient and present a synthesis of these together with our recommendations on how to select a delivery system when treating adult outpatients with asthma or COPD.

INHALED DELIVERY SYSTEMS

The characteristics, advantages, and limitations of the four broad types of delivery systems have been summarized extensively (10–14) (and chapters in this book). Not all drugs are available in each of the four device types, but most classes of therapy are, and often specific drugs and combinations are available in more than one device.

Characteristics of the different devices that may affect their selection are summarized in Tables 10.1 and 10.2. Devices differ in their size and portability. They also differ in the number of steps required to prepare them (15), in the force needed to load or actuate them (16), in the time taken to deliver the drug, and in the need for cleaning and maintenance, as well as in the inspiratory maneuver required to use them effectively (10). The number of steps has an impact on the ease of use and the likelihood that patients use the inhaler correctly (17). There are also quite significant differences in the carbon footprint of devices, reflecting whether or not they contain a propellant gas, what they are made from, how they are manufactured, and whether they can be reused or recycled. This is also an important consideration now for patients and payers in some countries (18, 19).

Devices differ in the proportion of drug delivered to the oropharynx and the large and small airways and this may influence clinicians' and patients' selection and use of a delivery system. Higher oropharyngeal deposition of corticosteroids increases the risk of local side effects which adversely affect adherence and persistence with therapy (26). The extent to which devices deliver drug particles to the peripheral airways compared to central airways has been claimed to affect the efficacy of therapy (27) but this is controversial (28). There is evidence that extra-fine particles act at the level of large- to moderate-caliber airways to produce most of their beneficial effect (29), and centrally deposited particles also affect peripheral airway function (30), suggesting central deposition is no less effective than peripheral deposition. However, it is possible that extra-fine formulations of ICS have greater effects on small airways than non-extra-fine formulations as a result of higher peripheral deposition (31), although it is possible that the differences are simply due to an overall increase in pulmonary deposition rather than greater delivery to small airways (32).

The availability of smart inhalers which incorporate sensors that detect the date and time of use, inspiratory flow, and inspired volume may also affect

Table 10.1: Summary of Device Features that May Affect Selection

Device Attributes	pMDI	SMI	DPI	Nebulizer
Portable	Yes	Yes	Yes	Jet - limited Ultrasonic - some
Need for loading	No	Initial insertion of cartridge - not for each dose	Some	Placing solution in chamber
Need for preparation before each dose	No If breath-actuated - yes	Yes	Yes	Yes
Manual force required for actuation (16)	High	Low	Medium to low	Very low
Need for coordination of actuation & inhalation	Yes If breath-actuated - no If spacer used - no	Minimal	No	No
Inspiratory maneuver	Slow and steady	Slow and steady	Hard and fast	Tidal breathing
Inspiratory effort required	Low	Low	Medium to high	Low
Carbon footprint	High	1/20th pMDI	1/10th pMDI	N/A
Oropharyngeal deposition	Low/medium	Low	Medium	Low
Time taken to deliver drug	Quick	Quick	Quick	Jet - slow Ultrasonic - quick
Regular cleaning recommended	Yes	No	No	Yes

Source: Data from (11–13, 15, 16, 21–25). Reprinted with Permission of the American Thoracic Society. Copyright © 2022 American Thoracic Society. All Rights Reserved. Halpin and Mahler (20). Annals of the American Thoracic Society Is an Official Journal of the American Thoracic Society).

Abbreviations: DPI = dry powder inhaler; PIFr = peak Inspiratory flow against simulated resistance; pMDI = pressurized metered-dose inhaler; SMI = slow mist inhaler.

device selection. These allow the identification of problems and feedback in real time (33) and can provide HCPs with objective data on adherence and technique (34, 35). They can be used as part of disease management programs to facilitate self-management (36) and may improve outcomes (37).

PATIENT FACTORS

A number of patient factors are relevant to inhaler device selection (Table 10.2). Patient's cognitive ability, their manual dexterity and coordination skills, the inspiratory flow that they can achieve, and their attitudes and beliefs are important factors when selecting a device. Poor inhaler technique and errors using devices are more common with advancing age (38), but this is likely to be

Table 10.2: **Summary of Factors Affecting Device Selection**

Device Attributes	Patient Factors	Clinician Factors
Molecule/drug class	Ability to perform	Knowledge of availability
Type of delivery system (pMDI,	conscious inhalation	of devices
DPI, SMI, nebulizer)	Cognitive ability	Familiarity with devices
Size	Manual dexterity	Personal preferences
Need for loading	Coordination	Availability of samples
Need for priming	Ability to perform correct	Formulary availability
Inspiratory maneuver required	inspiratory maneuver	Ease of teaching
Inspiratory effort required	PIFr	Desire to maintain
Carbon footprint	Familiarity with device	continuity of device
Ease of use	Attitudes and beliefs	
Pulmonary deposition		
Time taken to deliver drug		
Need for cleaning		
Smart features		
Cost		

Abbreviations: DPI = dry powder inhaler; PIFr = peak Inspiratory flow against simulated resistance; pMDI = pressurized metered-dose inhaler; SMI = slow mist inhaler.

mainly due to confounders such as cognitive impairment or reduced manual dexterity. When these factors have been independently assessed, older age alone has not been found to affect pMDI or DPI use (39, 40).

Cognitive impairment is not a common problem in patients with asthma but is found in 32–57% of COPD patients (41, 42). Adequate cognition is required to understand the instructions and perform the steps for preparing and using a handheld device or a nebulizer. Many patients with COPD and some with asthma have comorbidities that affect manual dexterity or grip strength, such as arthritis, neuromuscular or cerebral vascular disease. pMDIs require sufficient strength to actuate the inhaler, and although breath-actuated devices are triggered by inhalation they still require priming, which requires a degree of strength (16). Patients with poor dexterity may struggle to load a DPI, particularly if capsules require extraction from foil, insertion into the device, or puncturing prior to administration (16). Tremor may result in shaking of the device and of the dose (43). Loading of nebulizers and priming of SMIs can be performed in advance by a relative or carer if the patient is unable to perform these steps.

Adequate coordination is necessary to ensure the correct timing and sequence of exhaling completely, actuating the inhaler if necessary, inhaling in the correct manner, and then breath holding. With pMDIs, if the aerosol bolus is released too late in the respiratory maneuver, or if inspiration ceases on release of the aerosol, the lung deposition will be poor (44). Many patients lack coordination for the split-second timing required between beginning a slow inhalation and activation of a pMDI (45). SMIs are more tolerant of delay in inhalation as the plume duration is long (46), but premature inhalation will reduce drug delivery. Coordination is not needed for DPIs and nebulizers.

Inspiratory flow, flow acceleration, and inhaled volume are important factors for patients to successfully inhale drug particles from handheld devices into the lower respiratory tract (10). The recommended inspiratory flow is 30–60 L/min for a pMDI and 15–30 L/min for an SMI (47). Each DPI has a unique internal resistance and patients must create turbulent energy within the device during inhalation to disaggregate the powder into fine particles. Peak inspiratory flow (PIF), defined as the maximal airflow during a forced inspiratory maneuver, against the simulated resistance (r) of a specific DPI is a biomarker that can be used to assess whether a patient can achieve optimal drug deposition with that device (47). The minimal and optimal PIFr values required for effective use of DPIs differ between devices depending on their internal resistance. In general, for low to medium high-resistance DPIs, a minimal PIFr of 30 L/min and an optimal PIFr ≥ 60 L/min have been proposed (10, 48, 49). For a high-resistance DPI, a minimal PIFr of 20 L/min and an optimal PIFr ≥ 30 L/min have been proposed (49). Most patients with asthma can generate a sufficient PIFr to use all types of DPI (50), whereas in stable outpatient, with COPD, the prevalence of suboptimal PIFr (< 60 L/min) across low to medium high-resistance DPIs varied from 19% to 84% (51). Advanced age, female sex, and reduced inspiratory capacity (IC) but not FEV1 are the most consistent patient characteristics associated with a lower PIFr (51). In patients with COPD, age reduces PIFr independently of the severity of the disease (51, 52).

As well as physiological and physical factors, patients' beliefs and preferences must be taken into account when selecting an inhaled therapy (53). A key issue is familiarity with a device, and selecting a therapy in a device which the patient is already using may be the best strategy, provided they are using it correctly. Patients who are prescribed their preferred inhalation device have higher treatment satisfaction, fewer device use errors, better adherence, and lower health resource utilization and costs (54–57). A meta-analysis of patients' preferences regarding inhaler characteristics found that the common preferences were for small inhaler devices that were portable, durable, perceived as easy to use, and fast in medication administration (58). However, inhaler selection should take account of the individual patient's own preferences. Satisfaction with an inhaler device also affects compliance and persistence with inhaled therapy (59, 60).

CLINICIAN FACTORS

Clinicians' knowledge of the existence of different delivery systems, their familiarity with them, and their confidence about instructing patients on how to use them affect device selection (Table 10.2), but often their choice is based on habit (61). In some cases, selection is limited by availability of specific devices due to contractual or formulary limitations. New devices may take some time to appear on formularies and many formularies deliberately limit the number of different devices that are listed. Formularies may also deliberately restrict devices to specific classes such as pMDIs on the basis of cost and clinicians may be forced to prescribe a sub-optimal device for a specific patient. In some countries, particularly the USA, physicians are commonly provided with free samples of inhalers to give to their patients (62). Although allowing immediate initiation of therapy and demonstration of correct use of the device, the availability of samples will influence the choice of device. Continuing to prescribe a device which the patient is familiar with, and can use correctly, is important. In a Delphi analysis, most clinicians agreed that devices were not readily interchangeable, even if active substances and dosages were kept the same (63).

HCPs views on the desirable characteristics of devices and their ranking of importance differ significantly from those of patients (64), and nurses placed little importance on whether inhalers needed fine motor skills or hand strength (65). Ignoring these factors can clearly lead to inappropriate device selection.

Patients commonly make errors using devices (9, 66–68) and ease of teaching and assessment of correct inhaler technique are important attributes for clinicians when selecting an inhaler device (63). Many clinicians have limited knowledge about how to use inhalers, even those that have been in use for many years, with nearly 85% of HCPs unable to demonstrate the correct technique (69). Poor understanding of the correct use of devices also impacts the HCPs' ability to identify whether patients can use them properly, compromising appropriate device selection. Patient inhaler user technique is usually assessed by observing the patient using the device, sometimes using a checklist (70); however, this depends on the clinician knowing how the device should be used and recognizing critical errors. Observation of inhaler technique in a clinical setting may show that a patient knows how to use an inhaler, but gives no information about whether they do so on a regular basis (71).

SELECTING DEVICES FOR MAINTENANCE THERAPY COMPARED TO RELIEVER THERAPY

A different approach to selecting an inhaler device may needed when prescribing a once- or twice-daily maintenance therapy as compared to a reliever therapy which may be needed at any time of day as well as away from a patient's home. The size and portability of the delivery system are particularly important considerations when prescribing reliever medication.

INHALER-NAÏVE PATIENTS VERSUS THOSE ALREADY ON INHALED THERAPY

A different approach to selecting an inhaler device is needed when prescribing a device to a patient for the first time compared to prescribing a device to a patient who is already taking inhaled therapy. When selecting a device for the first time, the device should be selected on the basis of the characteristics discussed above using the approach outlined below. When adding or changing therapy in patients already using a device, if they have a good technique and are happy with the device, continuity of device should be the main determinant of the delivery system for the new therapy. COPD patients prescribed one or more additional inhaler devices requiring inhalation techniques similar to their previous device(s) showed better outcomes than those who were prescribed devices requiring different techniques (72), and switching of devices without a clinical justification has been associated with poorer outcomes (73). At follow-up review, a new delivery system may be needed if a new drug is required either as an alternative or as an addition and it is only available in a different device, or if the patient is unable or unwilling to use their current delivery system. When selecting a new delivery system in this setting, the characteristics discussed above using the approach outlined below should again be used to guide selection.

SELECTING A DELIVERY SYSTEM

A number of proposals on factors that should be considered when selecting an inhaler device have been published. However, until recently, there has been no attempt to analyze or reconcile these different perspectives. A systematic review of published algorithms for inhaler selection in outpatients with COPD identified nine different algorithms or hierarchical recommendations to guide clinicians with device selection in stable patients with COPD (4, 12, 13, 15, 18, 19, 51, 74, 75). The inclusion of the device, patient, and clinician factors discussed above and the order in which they were considered varied considerably between the different algorithms (Table 10.3) (20). The algorithm proposed by Janknegt et al. (15) is unique in that after three decision steps based on the patient's inhalation maneuver and inhalation strength, the device is then chosen according to a ranking of attributes including continuity of device, numbers

Table 10.3: Attributes and Factors Included in Published Algorithms for Inhaler Selection in Patients with COPD

Algorithm	Patient Factors									Device Attributes										HCP Factors					
	Age	Ability to perform conscious inhalation	Cognitive ability	Manual dexterity	Coordination	Ability to perform correct inspiratory manoeuvre	Inspiratory flow/PIFr	Familiarity with device	Personal preferences	Molecule/drug class	Type (pMDI, DPI, SMI, neb)	Size, robustness, and need for loading	Inspiratory effort required	Carbon footprint	Ease of use	Pulmonary deposition	Time taken to deliver drug	Smart features	Cost	Habit/preference	Knowledge	Availability of samples	Formulary	Ease of teaching	Continuity of device
Dekhuijzen (74, 77)	1				3		2																		
Dolovich (4)	2=				2	2=	2		8=	1		7			6=		6=		4	8=					5
Janknegt (15)	1					3					4*				4*								3		4*
Mahler (51)			1	2			3																		
Suarez-Barcelo † (13)			2=	2=	2=		1																		
Usmani ‡ (12)			1=	1=						2=		3=					3=		2=				2=	4	
Usmani (19)						1				3				2											
Virchow (18)						3								2											
Voshaar/Chapman (75, 76)	1#				2		3																		1

Source: Reprinted with Permission of the American Thoracic Society. Copyright © 2022 American Thoracic Society. All Rights Reserved. Halpin and Mahler (20) Annals of the American Thoracic Society Is an Official Journal of the American Thoracic Society.

Note: *Continuity of Device, Numbers of Steps Per Inhalation, Risk of (critical) Errors, Hygiene Aspects, a Feedback Mechanism, and Risk of Inhalation with an Empty Inhaler Were Incorporated in a System of Objectified Judgement Matrix. Numbers refer to rank order in which factors are considered by the respective authors.

† These Recommendations Are Specifically for Long-Term Care Settings. ‡ These Recommendations Are Specific for Elderly Patients.
# Ability to Perform Conscious Inhalation Is Included as the First Factor to Consider in the Original Algorithm Published by Voshaar et al. (75) but It Is Not Included in the English Version Published by Chapman et al. (76).

"=" = attributes given equal ranking in algorithm; DPI = dry powder inhaler; HCP = heath care professional; PIFr = peak inspiratory flow against simulated resistance; pMDI = pressurized metered-dose inhaler; SMI = soft mist inhaler.

Table 10.4: Questions to Guide Selection of Inhaler Delivery System

Patient Factors

- Can the patient perform a specific inspiratory effort? (incorporates cognitive and respiratory muscle functions)
- Can the patient handle/use the device? (considers manual dexterity and hand strength)
- If a DPI is considered: Can the patient generate an optimal peak inspiratory flow? (measured against the simulated resistance of the specific DPI)

Device Attribute

- Is the molecule(s)/drug class available in the device?

HCP Factor

- Is the patient currently on inhaled therapy and able to use their current device correctly, and if so, can new therapy be prescribed in the same device?

Source: Originally published in: Halpin and Mahler with Permission.
Abbreviation: DPI = dry powder inhaler.

of steps per inhalation, risk of errors, hygiene aspects, a feedback mechanism, and risk of inhalation with an empty inhaler. These factors were incorporated in an objectified judgement matrix which ranks inhalers, but the decision is not patient specific.

Given the numerous medication-device options available for the treatment of asthma and COPD, there is a clear need for practical information to assist HCPs in selecting an inhaler delivery system. A systematic approach to inhaler selection seems better than the current "gestalt" by clinicians, but no rigorous assessment of any of the published algorithms has been performed. The systematic review of algorithms for inhaler selection in COPD found that patient factors were considered most frequently in the algorithms (19 times) compared with device attributes (10 times) and HCP factors (7 times). On the basis of the frequency of their appearance in the algorithms, five specific attributes/factors were identified as key factors for device selection: ability to perform the required inspiratory maneuver and handle the device correctly, sufficient inspiratory flow for dry powder inhalers, availability of molecule(s) in the device, and continuity of device (Table 10.4) (20).

When recommending an inhaled therapy, the first question to consider is whether or not the patient is already using an inhaler device, and if so, whether they are using it correctly (Figure 10.1). If the answer to both of these questions is yes, then continuity of device should be the overriding principle guiding the choice of the new therapy. If a patient is not currently taking an inhaled therapy, if there are problems with their ability to use their current device, or if a change of drug requires the use of a different device because the new treatment is not available in the same device, then a stepwise approach to selecting the optimum device is required.

Selecting a device that contains the required drug or class of drug seems the next most logical step and availability of the device in a formulary must be the next consideration. HCPs must then make a provisional choice of device taking into account their own beliefs and habits as well as those of the patient. This should include patient's preferences on size and portability, need for loading, strength required, time taken to deliver the drug, efficiency of drug deposition, ability of the HCP to teach its correct use, cost, and carbon footprint.

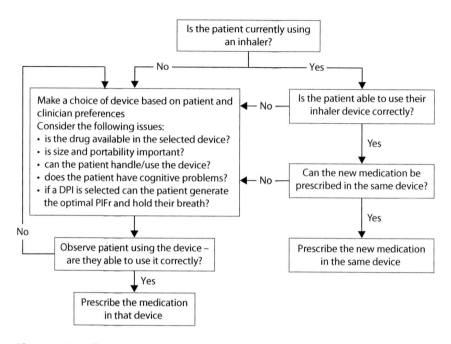

Figure 10.1 Recommended approach to selecting an inhaler delivery system. DPI = dry powder inhaler; PIFr = peak inspiratory flow against simulated resistance.

If the provisional choice is a pMDI, many clinicians recommend that a valved holding chamber (spacer) should always be used to minimize the difficulties patients have with coordination and performing the optimal inspiratory maneuver for a pMDI, as well as increasing pulmonary and reducing oropharyngeal deposition. This is particularly important for corticosteroid-containing pMDIs (10) but is also relevant to optimize the delivery of bronchodilators. Currently available spacers range in volume from <50–750 mL (78) but spacers with volumes from 150 to 250 mL have been shown to be as effective as those with larger volumes (79) and are more portable. Retrospective analysis of primary care records in the UK found significantly more patients prescribed ICS via a pMDI and a spacer were controlled compared with those on pMDIs alone (80); however, a similar but larger analysis with matching of patient characteristics found no evidence that prescribing spacer devices was associated with improved asthma outcomes or reduced oropharyngeal candidiasis (81). If there is any doubt that the patient will not be able to use a pMDI correctly, they should be prescribed a spacer; however, there is evidence that incorrect use of pMDIs is more common in older patients if they use a spacer (82). It has been suggested that each pairing of a pMDI device plus spacer should be considered as a unique delivery system and that once a spacer has been chosen, like the device itself, it should not be changed without good reason (83).

The selection of a provisional device should also take account of the patient's cognitive ability and manual dexterity. For those with impaired cognition, Dekhuijzen et al. (53, 74, 77) recommend two options for an inhaler delivery system: a pMD onI + spacer or nebulizer therapy. Similarly, Suarez-Barcelo et al. (13) suggest pMDI + spacer, SMI, and nebulizer as options for those with "moderate/severe cognitive impairment." For individuals with poor manual dexterity, Mahler (51) proposed nebulizer therapy as the preferred delivery system, while Suarez-Barcelo et al. (13) suggested a nebulizer be "a device to consider" along with pMDI + spacer or SMI for those with "insufficient dexterity." Selecting the provisional device could be assisted by using a decision aid (84, 85).

Once a provisional device has been selected, the patient's ability to use the device correctly should be assessed. This includes checking that they load and prime the device correctly, adequately coordinate inhalation with actuation, and perform the correct inspiratory maneuver. If the provisional device is a DPI, clinicians should objectively assess the patient's ability to generate sufficient inspiratory flow by measuring their PIFr. If the patient has a suboptimal PIF as defined by < 60 L/minute, or < 30 L/minute for a high-resistance DPI, Voshaar, Dekhuijzen, Suarez-Barcelo, Mahler and Janknegt, (13, 15, 51, 74, 75, 77) all propose that a pMDI, SMI, or a nebulizer be prescribed instead. As well as assessing the PIFr, clinicians should check that the patient is able to hold their breath for at least 5 seconds after performing the inhalation, as some patients may be able to generate the desired PIFr, but they then find it hard to hold their breath as a result of the excessive use of all the respiratory muscles and the discomfort of breathing.

If the patient can use the provisional device satisfactorily then this should be the device that is prescribed, but if they cannot, an alternative provisional device should be selected and the patient's ability to use this device is correctly assessed. This iterative approach should continue until a device that can be used correctly is identified.

CONCLUSION

A systematic approach which takes account of device characteristics and patient and clinician factors should be used to select the optimum delivery system for each patient.

REFERENCES

1. Global Initiative for Chronic Obstructive Lung Disease (GOLD). Global strategy for the diagnosis, management, and prevention of chronic obstructive pulmonary disease. 2021 Report. [cited 2021 Jan 11]. Available from: http://www.goldcopd.org/
2. Nici L, Mammen MJ, Charbek E, et al. Pharmacologic management of chronic obstructive pulmonary disease. An Official American Thoracic Society Clinical Practice Guideline. Am J Respir Crit Care Med 2020;201(9):e56–e69.
3. Global Initiative for Asthma. Global strategy for asthma management and prevention. (updated 2019). 2019. Available from: http://www.ginasthma.org
4. Dolovich MB, Ahrens RC, Hess DR, et al. Device selection and outcomes of aerosol therapy: Evidence-based guidelines: American College of Chest Physicians/American College of Asthma, Allergy, and Immunology. Chest 2005;127(1):335–371.
5. Wilson SR, Strub P, Buist AS, et al. Shared treatment decision making improves adherence and outcomes in poorly controlled asthma. Am J Respir Crit Care Med 2010;181(6):566–577.
6. Inhaler Error Steering Committee, Price D, Bosnic-Anticevich S, et al. Inhaler competence in asthma: Common errors, barriers to use and recommended solutions. Respir Med 2013;107(1):37–46.

7. Capstick T, Atack K. The leeds inhaler device guide. 2018. [cited 2021 April]. Available from: http://www.cpwy.org/doc/2003.pdf

8. Hanania NA, Braman S, Adams SG, et al. The role of inhalation delivery devices in COPD: Perspectives of patients and health care providers. Chronic Obstr Pulm Dis 2018;5(2):111–123.

9. Sanchis J, Gich I, Pedersen S. Systematic review of errors in inhaler use: Has patient technique improved over time? Chest 2016;150(2):394–406.

10. Laube BL, Janssens HM, de Jongh FH, et al. What the pulmonary specialist should know about the new inhalation therapies. Eur Respir J 2011;37(6):1308–1331.

11. Sanchis J, Corrigan C, Levy ML, et al. Inhaler devices - from theory to practice. Respir Med 2013;107(4):495–502.

12. Usmani OS. Choosing the right inhaler for your asthma or COPD patient. Ther Clin Risk Manag 2019;15:461–472.

13. Suarez-Barcelo M, Micca JL, Clackum S, et al. Chronic obstructive pulmonary disease in the long-term care setting: Current practices, challenges, and unmet needs. Curr Opin Pulm Med 2017;23(Suppl 1):S1–S28.

14. Capstick TG, Clifton IJ. Inhaler technique and training in people with chronic obstructive pulmonary disease and asthma. Expert Rev Respir Med 2012;6(1):91–101; quiz 2–3.

15. Janknegt R, Kooistra J, Metting E, et al. Rational selection of inhalation devices in the treatment of chronic obstructive pulmonary disease by means of the System of Objectified Judgement Analysis (SOJA). Eur J Hosp Pharm 2021;28(2):e4.

16. Ciciliani A-M, Langguth P, Wachtel H. Handling forces for the use of different inhaler devices. Int J Pharm 2019;560:315–321.

17. Klijn SL, Hiligsmann M, Evers S, et al. Effectiveness and success factors of educational inhaler technique interventions in asthma & COPD patients: A systematic review. NPJ Prim Care Respir Med 2017;27(1):24.

18. Virchow JC, Crompton GK, Dal Negro R, et al. Importance of inhaler devices in the management of airway disease. Respir Med 2008;102(1):10–19.

19. Usmani O, Capstick T, Saleem A, et al. Inhaler choice guideline. 2020. Available from: https://www.guidelines.co.uk/respiratory/inhaler-choice-guideline/455503.article

20. Halpin DMG, Mahler DA. A systematic review of published algorithms for selecting an inhaled delivery system in COPD. Ann Am Thorac Soc 2022;19(7):1213–1220.

21. Dhand R, Dolovich M, Chipps B, et al. The role of nebulized therapy in the management of COPD: Evidence and recommendations. COPD 2012;9(1):58–72.

22. Panigone S, Sandri F, Ferri R, et al. Environmental impact of inhalers for respiratory diseases: Decreasing the carbon footprint while preserving patient-tailored treatment. BMJ Open Respir Res 2020;7(1):e000571.

23. Hänsel M, Bambach T, Wachtel H. Reduced environmental impact of the reusable Respimat® Soft Mist™ inhaler compared with pressurised metered-dose inhalers. Adv Ther 2019;36(9):2487–2492.

24. Fink JB, Colice GL, Hodder R. Inhaler devices for patients with COPD. COPD 2013;10(4):523–535.

25. Dolovich MB, Dhand R. Aerosol drug delivery: Developments in device design and clinical use. Lancet 2011;377(9770):1032–1045.

26. Molimard M, Le Gros V, Robinson P, et al. Prevalence and associated factors of oropharyngeal side effects in users of inhaled corticosteroids in a real-life setting. J Aerosol Med Pulm Drug Deliv 2010;23(2):91–95.

27. Postma DS, Roche N, Colice G, et al. Comparing the effectiveness of small-particle versus large-particle inhaled corticosteroid in COPD. Int J Chron Obstruct Pulmon Dis 2014;9:1163–1186.

28. Lavorini F, Pedersen S, Usmani OS. Dilemmas, confusion, and misconceptions related to small airways directed therapy. Chest 2017;151(6):1345–1355.

29. Boulet LP. Comparative improvement of asthma symptoms and expiratory flows after corticosteroid treatment: A method to assess the effect of corticosteroids on large vs. small airways? Respir Med 2006;100(3):496–502.

30. Timmins SC, Diba C, Schoeffel RE, et al. Changes in oscillatory impedance and nitrogen washout with combination fluticasone/salmeterol therapy in COPD. Respir Med 2014;108(2):344–350.

31. Goldin JG, Tashkin DP, Kleerup EC, et al. Comparative effects of hydrofluoroalkane and chlorofluorocarbon beclomethasone dipropionate inhalation on small airways: Assessment with functional helical thin-section computed tomography. J Allergy Clin Immunol 1999;104(6):S258–S267.

32. Busse WW, Brazinsky S, Jacobson K, et al. Efficacy response of inhaled beclomethasone dipropionate in asthma is proportional to dose and is improved by formulation with a new propellant. J Allergy Clin Immunol 1999;104(6):1215–1222.

33. Carpenter DM, Roberts CA, Sage AJ, et al. A review of electronic devices to assess inhaler technique. Curr Allergy Asthma Rep 2017;17(3):17.

34. Chan AH, Harrison J, Black PN, et al. Using electronic monitoring devices to measure inhaler adherence: A practical guide for clinicians. J Allergy Clin Immunol Pract 2015;3(3):335–349 e1-5.

35. Bowler R, Allinder M, Jacobson S, et al. Real-world use of rescue inhaler sensors, electronic symptom questionnaires and physical activity monitors in COPD. BMJ Open Respir Res 2019;6(1):e000350.

36. Halpin D, Banks L, Martello A. Working together to go 'beyond the pill': Building a virtuous network of collaborators. BMJ Innov 2016;2(1):1.

37. Price D, Jones R, Pfister P, et al. Maximizing adherence and gaining new information for your chronic obstructive pulmonary disease (MAGNIFY COPD): Study protocol for the pragmatic, cluster randomized trial evaluating the impact of dual bronchodilator with add-on sensor and electronic monitoring on clinical outcomes. Pragmat Obs Res 2021;12:25–35.

38. Barbara S, Kritikos V, Bosnic-Anticevich S. Inhaler technique: Does age matter? A systematic review. Eur Respir Rev 2017;26(146):170055.

39. Gray SL, Williams DM, Pulliam CC, et al. Characteristics predicting incorrect metered-dose inhaler technique in older subjects. Arch Intern Med 1996;156(9):984–988.

40. Maricoto T, Santos D, Carvalho C, et al. Assessment of poor inhaler technique in older patients with asthma or COPD: A predictive tool for clinical risk and inhaler performance. Drugs Aging 2020;37(8):605–616.

41. Yohannes AM, Chen W, Moga AM, et al. Cognitive impairment in chronic obstructive pulmonary disease and chronic heart failure: A systematic review and meta-analysis of observational studies. J Am Med Dir Assoc 2017;18(5):451 e1–e11.

42. Cleutjens FA, Franssen FM, Spruit MA, et al. Domain-specific cognitive impairment in patients with COPD and control subjects. Int J Chron Obstruct Pulmon Dis 2017;12:1–11.

43. Barrons R, Pegram A, Borries A. Inhaler device selection: Special considerations in elderly patients with chronic obstructive pulmonary disease. Am J Health Syst Pharm 2011;68(13):1221–1232.

44. Newman SP, Pavia D, Clarke SW. How should a pressurized beta-adrenergic bronchodilator be inhaled? Eur J Respir Dis 1981;62(1):3–21.

45. McFadden ER, Jr. Improper patient techniques with metered dose inhalers: Clinical consequences and solutions to misuse. J Allergy Clin Immunol 1995;96(2):278–283.

46. Keating GM. Tiotropium Respimat((R)) Soft Mist inhaler: A review of its use in chronic obstructive pulmonary disease. Drugs 2014;74(15):1801–1816.

47. Mahler DA, Halpin DMG. Peak inspiratory flow as a predictive therapeutic biomarker in COPD. Chest 2021;160(2):491–498.

48. Ghosh S, Ohar JA, Drummond MB. Peak inspiratory flow rate in chronic obstructive pulmonary disease: Implications for dry powder inhalers. J Aerosol Med Pulm Drug Deliv 2017;30:381–387.

49. Haidl P, Heindl S, Siemon K, et al. Inhalation device requirements for patients' inhalation maneuvers. Respir Med 2016;118:65–75.

50. Haughney J, Lee AJ, McKnight E, et al. Peak inspiratory flow measured at different inhaler resistances in patients with asthma. J Allergy Clin Immunol Pract 2021;9(2):890–896.

51. Mahler DA. The role of inspiratory flow in selection and use of inhaled therapy for patients with chronic obstructive pulmonary disease. Respir Med 2020;161:105857.

52. Jarvis S, Ind PW, Shiner RJ. Inhaled therapy in elderly COPD patients: Time for re-evaluation? Age Ageing 2007;36(2):213–218.

53. Dekhuijzen PN, Lavorini F, Usmani OS. Patients' perspectives and preferences in the choice of inhalers: The case for Respimat® or HandiHaler®. Patient Prefer Adherence 2016;10:1561–1572.

54. Chorao P, Pereira AM, Fonseca JA. Inhaler devices in asthma and COPD– an assessment of inhaler technique and patient preferences. Respir Med 2014;108(7):968–975.

55. Oliveira MVC, Pizzichini E, da Costa CH, et al. Evaluation of the preference, satisfaction and correct use of Breezhaler((R)) and Respimat((R)) inhalers in patients with chronic obstructive pulmonary disease - INHALATOR study. Respir Med 2018;144:61–67.

56. Dahl R, Kaplan A. A systematic review of comparative studies of tiotropium Respimat(R) and tiotropium HandiHaler(R) in patients with chronic obstructive pulmonary disease: Does inhaler choice matter? BMC Pulm Med 2016;16(1):135.

57. Chrystyn H, Small M, Milligan G, et al. Impact of patients' satisfaction with their inhalers on treatment compliance and health status in COPD. Respir Med 2014;108(2):358–365.

58. Navaie M, Dembek C, Cho-Reyes S, et al. Inhaler device feature preferences among patients with obstructive lung diseases: A systematic review and meta-analysis. Medicine 2020;99(25):e20718.

59. Schurmann W, Schmidtmann S, Moroni P, et al. Respimat Soft Mist inhaler versus hydrofluoroalkane metered dose inhaler: Patient preference and satisfaction. Treat Respir Med 2005;4(1):53–61.

60. Barbosa CD, Balp MM, Kulich K, et al. A literature review to explore the link between treatment satisfaction and adherence, compliance, and persistence. Patient Prefer Adherence 2012;6:39–48.

61. Halpin DMG. Understanding irrationality: The key to changing behaviours and improving management of respiratory diseases? Lancet Respir Med 2018;6(10):737–739.

62. Brown JD, Doshi PA, Talbert JC. Utilization of free medication samples in the United States in a nationally representative sample: 2009–2013. Res Social Adm Pharm 2017;13(1):193–200.

63. Ninane V, Brusselle GG, Louis R, et al. Usage of inhalation devices in asthma and chronic obstructive pulmonary disease: A Delphi consensus statement. Expert Opin Drug Deliv 2014;11(3):313–323.

64. Roche N, Scheuch G, Pritchard JN, et al. Patient focus and regulatory considerations for inhalation device design: Report from the 2015 IPAC-RS/ ISAM workshop. J Aerosol Med Pulm Drug Deliv 2017;30(1):1–13.

65. Bogelund M, Hagelund L, Asmussen MB. COPD-treating nurses' preferences for inhaler attributes - a discrete choice experiment. Curr Med Res Opin 2017;33(1):71–75.

66. Melani AS, Bonavia M, Cilenti V, et al. Inhaler mishandling remains common in real life and is associated with reduced disease control. Respir Med 2011;105(6):930–938.

67. Molimard M, Raherison C, Lignot S, et al. Chronic obstructive pulmonary disease exacerbation and inhaler device handling: Real-life assessment of 2935 patients. Eur Respir J 2017;49(2):1601794.

68. Alhaddad B, Smith FJ, Robertson T, et al. Patients' practices and experiences of using nebuliser therapy in the management of COPD at home. BMJ Open Respir Res 2015;2(1):e000076.

69. Plaza V, Giner J, Rodrigo GJ, et al. Errors in the use of inhalers by health care professionals: A systematic review. J Allergy Clin Immunol Pract 2018;6(3):987–995.

70. Batterink J, Dahri K, Aulakh A, et al. Evaluation of the use of inhaled medications by hospital inpatients with chronic obstructive pulmonary disease. Can J Hosp Pharm 2012;65(2):111–118.

71. Pritchard JN, Nicholls C. Emerging technologies for electronic monitoring of adherence, inhaler competence, and true adherence. J Aerosol Med Pulm Drug Deliv 2015;28(2):69–81.

72. Bosnic-Anticevich S, Chrystyn H, Costello RW, et al. The use of multiple respiratory inhalers requiring different inhalation techniques has an adverse effect on COPD outcomes. Int J Chron Obstruct Pulmon Dis 2017;12:59–71.

73. Thomas M, Price D, Chrystyn H, et al. Inhaled corticosteroids for asthma: Impact of practice level device switching on asthma control. BMC Pulm Med 2009;9:1.

74. Dekhuijzen PN. [Inhaler therapy for adults with obstructive lung diseases: Powder or aerosol?]. Ned Tijdschr Geneeskd 1998;142(24) :1369–1374. Dutch

75. Voshaar T, App EM, Berdel D, et al. [Recommendations for the choice of inhalatory systems for drug prescription]. Pneumologie 2001;55(12): 579–586. German.

76. Chapman KR, Voshaar TH, Virchow JC. Inhaler choice in primary practice. Eur Respir Rev 2005;14:117–122.

77. Dekhuijzen PN, Vincken W, Virchow JC, et al. Prescription of inhalers in asthma and COPD: Towards a rational, rapid and effective approach. Respir Med 2013;107(12):1817–1821.

78. Newman SP. Spacer devices for metered dose inhalers. Clin Pharmacokinet 2004;43(6):349–360.

79. Mitchell JP, Nagel MW. Valved holding chambers (VHCs) for use with pressurised metered-dose inhalers (pMDIs): A review of causes of inconsistent medication delivery. Prim Care Respir J 2007;16(4):207–214.

80. Levy ML, Hardwell A, McKnight E, et al. Asthma patients' inability to use a pressurised metered-dose inhaler (pMDI) correctly correlates with poor asthma control as defined by the global initiative for asthma (GINA) strategy: A retrospective analysis. Prim Care Respir J 2013;22(4):406–411.

81. Guilbert TW, Colice G, Grigg J, et al. Real-life outcomes for patients with asthma prescribed spacers for use with either extrafine- or fine-particle inhaled corticosteroids. J Allergy Clin Immunol Pract 2017;5(4):1040–1049, e4.

82. Ho SF, OMahony MS, Steward JA, et al. Inhaler technique in older people in the community. Age Ageing 2004;33(2):185–188.

83. McIvor RA, Devlin HM, Kaplan A. Optimizing the delivery of inhaled medication for respiratory patients: The role of valved holding chambers. Can Respir J 2018;2018:5076259.

84. Gagné ME, Légaré F, Moisan J, et al. Development of a patient decision aid on inhaled corticosteroids use for adults with asthma. J Asthma 2016;53(9):964–974.

85. Stacey D, Légaré F, Lewis K, et al. Decision aids for people facing health treatment or screening decisions. Cochrane Database Syst Rev 2017;4(4):CD001431.

11 Inhalation Therapy in the Intensive Care Unit

Jie Li and Rajiv Dhand

CONTENTS

INTRODUCTION

More than five million patients are admitted annually to U.S. Intensive Care Units (ICUs) (1). Many patients admitted to ICUs require intensive or invasive monitoring, support of airway, breathing, or circulation, and stabilization of acute or life-threatening medical problems. ICU patients often require respiratory support, such as oxygen (low and high flow) by mask or nasal cannula, and ventilatory support, such as noninvasive ventilation (NIV), or invasive mechanical ventilation (IMV), to help them breathe and maintain oxygenation. Inhaled therapies, especially bronchodilators, corticosteroids, and antibiotics, are commonly prescribed in patients receiving care in the ICU (2, 3). Many patients who require aerosol therapy in the ICU setting have chronic respiratory problems and have been receiving aerosolized medications prior to admission. Devices employed in ambulatory patients, including pressurized metered-dose inhalers (pMDIs), dry powder inhalers (DPIs), soft mist inhalers (SMIs), and small-volume nebulizers (SVNs), are not designed and approved for aerosol administration in patients receiving respiratory support by IMV, NIV, or high-flow nasal cannula (HFNC). Thus, the challenge of administering aerosolized therapies is to adapt these aerosol-generating devices to the equipment employed for patients requiring various modes of respiratory support in the ICU.

Clinicians taking care of patients requiring respiratory support with IMV, NIV, or HFNC in the ICU have the choice to either interrupt these therapies and administer aerosols with the techniques employed in ambulatory patients, or to integrate these aerosol-generators into the respiratory support equipment and provide effective targeted dosing to the lung, with minimal disruption of respiratory and ventilatory support (4, 5). Discontinuing the respiratory support may cause precipitous drops in oxygenation, alveolar collapse, increased work of breathing, cardiovascular instability, and dyspnea. Given the harm of interrupting respiratory support to administer conventional inhalation therapy for these patients in the ICU, aerosolized medications need to be delivered in conjunction with respiratory support. However, simply plugging an aerosol device into an oxygen or ventilator circuit is not straightforward and may impact delivery efficiency as well as patient safety. For example, an SVN connected to a ventilator circuit for intubated patients delivered <25% of the lung dose achieved in spontaneously breathing non-intubated patients (6). For medications whose actions are dependent on an adequate lung dose for effects, such as

DOI: 10.1201/9781003269014-11

Ventilator-related
• Ventilation mode
• Tidal volume
• Respiratory rate
• Duty cycle
• Inspiratory waveform
• Breath-triggering mechanism

Device-related–pMDI
• Type of spacer or adapter
• Position of spacer in circuit
• Timing of pMDI actuation
• Type of pMDI

Drug-related
• Dose
• Formulation
• Aerosol particle size
• Targeted site for delivery
• Duration of action

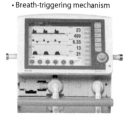
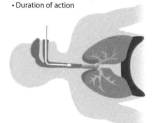

Patient Wye

Clear Chamber
AeroChamber* H.C.
MIDI Actuator

AeroChamber*
H.C. M.V.
Connector

Inspiratory
Limb

Circuit-related
• Endotracheal or tracheostomy tube
• Humidity of inhaled gas
• Density of inhaled gas
• Leak in circuit
• Bias flow

Device-related–Nebulizer
• Type of nebulizer
• Fill volume
• Gas flow rate
• Cycling: inspiration vs. continuous
• Duration of nebulization
• Position in circuit

Patient-related
• Severity of airway obstruction
• Mechanism of airway obstruction
• Presence of dynamic hyperinflation
• Patient-ventilator synchrony

Figure 11.1 Factors influencing aerosol delivery in patients receiving invasive mechanical ventilation. pMDI = pressurized metered-dose inhaler.

antibiotics, surfactants, and muco-active agents, a goal of aerosol administration to patients in the ICU is to achieve or exceed the target dose levels achieved with the drug label in the ambulatory patient (7).

Aerosol devices are not designed for use in a pressurized environment, and inserting them into pressurized circuits may cause leaks, reduce circuit pressure, and negatively impact gas volumes delivered to patients. The optimal techniques for aerosol therapy in patients in the ICU differ from those employed in ambulatory patients and require appropriate device selection, placement, operation, and dose administration (volume or frequency of drug delivery) (8).

AEROSOL GENERATORS AND THEIR CONFIGURATION FOR ICU PATIENTS

Considerable research, from bench to bedside, has focused on identifying factors impacting aerosol delivery during IMV(Figure 11.1), NIV (Figure 11.2), and HFNC (9–11). Variables associated with aerosol therapy during mechanical ventilation, first presented by Dhand and Tobin (12), have become a blueprint for assessing aerosol administration for a broader range of respiratory support. Aerosol delivery effectiveness is influenced by not only patient characteristics, such as the inhalation technique and severity of airway disease, but also the characteristics of aerosol devices integrated into respiratory support devices, their placement in the circuit, and the interface of these devices to patients (12, 13). As such, the features of aerosol devices that are commonly employed for aerosol delivery in the ICU, as well as a host of factors influencing aerosol delivery via each type of respiratory support (IMV, NIV, and HFNC), will be reviewed (Table 11.1), and considerations for optimal aerosol delivery will be summarized in this chapter (Table 11.2).

Devices Employed for Aerosol Delivery in the ICU

Nebulizers are the most utilized aerosol devices in the ICU. The advantages of nebulizers include little to no requirement for coordination of breathing patterns or inspiratory effort, the ability to deliver a wide range of liquid medications,

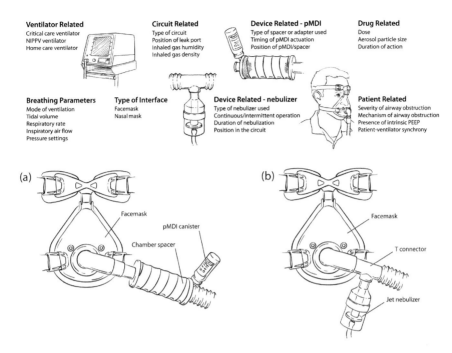

Ventilator Related
Critical care ventilator
NIPPV ventilator
Home care ventilator

Circuit Related
Type of circuit
Position of leak port
Inhaled gas humidity
Inhaled gas density

Device Related - pMDI
Type of spacer or adapter used
Timing of pMDI actuation
Position of pMDI/spacer

Drug Related
Dose
Aerosol particle size
Duration of action

Breathing Parameters
Mode of ventilation
Tidal volume
Respiratory rate
Inspiratory air flow
Pressure settings

Type of Interface
Facemask
Nasal mask

Device Related - nebulizer
Type of nebulizer used
Continuous/intermittent operation
Duration of nebulization
Position in the circuit

Patient Related
Severity of airway obstruction
Mechanism of airway obstruction
Presence of intrinsic PEEP
Patient-ventilator synchrony

(a) Facemask / pMDI canister / Chamber spacer

(b) Facemask / T connector / Jet nebulizer

Figure 11.2 Factors influencing aerosol delivery in patients receiving noninvasive ventilation (top panel). The connection of pMDIs and nebulizers with facemasks is shown in the Bottom panel. pMDI = pressurized metered-dose inhaler. *Abbreviations*: NIPPV = non invasive positive pressure ventilation; PEEP = positive end- expiratory pressure; pMDI = pressurized metered-dose inhaler.

and the relative ease of adjusting the administered dose placed in the reservoir (14). Nebulizers can be attached to a ventilator circuit with commonly available T-adapters. The spring-loaded T-adapter obviates the need for disconnecting the circuit for each nebulizer treatment (Figure 11.3).

A pMDI consisting of a canister and mouthpiece actuator is open to the atmosphere and cannot be directly used in a pressurized circuit. When a pMDI is used in-line with a pressurized circuit, the drug canister is removed from the actuator and used with a third-party spacer or adapter (Figure 11.3). When a pMDI is actuated, large particles containing propellants, preservatives, and medication, are emitted at high velocity and become smaller and slower as they traverse the first 10 cm. The use of a reservoir device allows propellants to evaporate, reduces particle size, slows down the velocity of the aerosol particles, and decreases impactive deposition as the aerosol passes into the circuit (14). Synchronizing pMDI actuation with the start of inspiration is critical for efficient drug delivery during ventilation, as random actuation greatly reduces the inhaled dose (15).

The SMI uses mechanical energy to create low-velocity and small particle size aerosols of 10 μl of liquid solutions in a single actuation lasting 1.2 seconds. Again, the SMI is designed to be open to the atmosphere and requires a third-party adapter to be used in ventilator circuits. There is great variability between different adapters. A reservoir may be used but is not critical for the use of SMI in which emitted particles are smaller than the pMDI. Because each actuation emits aerosol for 1.2 seconds (14), inspiratory time should match the duration of

Table 11.1: Variables that Affect Aerosol Delivery and Deposition during Various Modes of Respiratory Support in the ICU

Variables		HFNC	NIV	IMV
Differences	Interfaces	Size of nasal cannula, connection tightness of nasal cannula	Vented vs non-vented mask, nasal mask vs full face mask vs total face mask vs helmet	The size of artificial airway, endotracheal tube vs tracheostomy
	Settings	Gas flows	Modes, pressure settings	Mode, ventilation parameters including tidal volume, respiratory rate, duty cycle, trigger mechanism, and inspiratory flow waveform
	Others	Open mouth vs close mouth breathing	Leak; single limb vs dual limb ventilator	Patient-ventilator synchrony
Common	Patient related	Severity and mechanism of airway obstruction, presence of dynamic hyperinflation		
	Aerosol device related	pMDI: type and volume of third-party spacer or adapter, the position of the spacer in the circuit, timing of actuation. Nebulizer: type and placement of nebulizer, fill volume, inspiration synchronized vs continuous, duration of nebulization, driving gas flow		
	Circuit related	Humidification, circuit leak		
	Drug related	Dose, formulation, aerosol particle size, targeted site for delivery, duration of action		

Abbreviations: HFNC = high-flow nasal cannula; IMV = invasive mechanical ventilation; NIV = noninvasive ventilation; pMDI = pressurized metered dose inhaler.

aerosol emission, and gas flow from the ventilator should be synchronized with SMI actuation.

DPIs are passive devices that require patients to generate an inspiration flow, usually >30 L/min, to draw the powder from the reservoir (14). In the ICU environment, the DPI cannot be integrated into a circuit, and there are no approved commercially available methods for DPI administration during ventilator support. In addition, the powders can be greatly affected by humidity, which causes the powder to clump and reduces the dispersion of the drug into respirable particles (16).

Configuration of Inhalation Devices in ICU Patients

The configuration of medical aerosol inhalation devices for patients in ICUs depends on the medication, device availability with those drugs, the respiratory support device being used (Table 11.3), and whether the patient could tolerate interruption of respiratory support.

Table 11.2: Optimization of Aerosol Delivery during Various Modes of Respiratory Support in the ICU

		HFNC	NIV	IMV
Interface		Large size of nasal cannula and tightly connect it to patient nasal prongs	Non-vented mask is preferred	Changing artificial airway size or type for the sole purpose of improving aerosol delivery is not recommended
Aerosol device		VMN or pMDI with spacer are preferred, pMDI needs to be actuated at the beginning of inspiration		
Aerosol device position	VMN	At the inlet of humidifier	Between mask and exhalation valve in the single-limb ventilator and between mask and Y-piece in the dual-limb ventilator	At the inlet of humidifier
	pMDI and spacer	Close to nasal cannula		Close to Y-piece in the inspiratory limb
Humidification		No need to turn off humidifier	Humidification does not affect aerosol delivery	Turning off humidifier for routine aerosol therapy is not recommended
Settings		Titrate flow down during aerosol delivery	Changing the mode or settings for the sole purpose of improving aerosol delivery is not recommended	

Abbreviations: HFNC = high-flow nasal cannula; IMV = invasive mechanical ventilation; NIV = noninvasive ventilation; pMDI = pressurized metered dose inhaler; VMN = vibrating mesh nebulizer.

If patients are placed on invasive mechanical ventilation, interruption of ventilation is not recommended for aerosol administration. The aerosol device must be placed in-line with the ventilator. Besides nebulizers, pMDIs can be placed in-line with a spacer or adapter to deliver aerosolized medication (Figure 11.3). On the other hand, some patients receiving NIV or HFNC may tolerate interruption of therapy for short intervals to provide aerosol delivery, such as individual actuation of pMDIs or SMIs. Interruption for 10–15 minutes to provide nebulizer treatments may not be as well tolerated. In patients requiring consistent NIV or HFNC, an interruption of respiratory support could have greater adverse effects than the potential benefit of aerosol administration. Fortunately, using optimal techniques to administer aerosols via NIV or HFNC can produce similar inhaled doses and clinical effects as conventional aerosol devices (10, 11). Thus, interrupting NIV or HFNC for the sole purpose of improving aerosol delivery efficiency creates undue risk for patients. Nevertheless, an assessment of risks vs benefits should guide the decision whether to interrupt NIV or HFNC to administer conventional nebulization via mouthpiece or facemask, or to place a nebulizer in-line with NIV or HFNC.

Some aerosolized medications have a short half-life, requiring continuous administration, such as inhaled epoprostenol for patients with severe

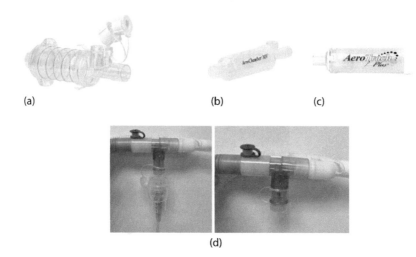

(a)   (b)   (c)

(d)

Figure 11.3 Adapters used to connect pressurized metered-dose inhalers (pMDIs) and nebulizers in-line in ventilator circuits. Reservoir chambers used to connect pMDIs in mechanically ventilated patients are shown (top panel, a and b). A special adapter is employed to connect pMDIs to tracheostomy tubes (c). A jet nebulizer is placed in-line with the ventilator circuit via a spring-loaded T-adapter (d, left). When the nebulization is completed, the jet nebulizer is removed from the ventilator circuit, leaving the T-adapter in-line with the Port capped (d, right).

Table 11.3: Characteristics of Aerosol Delivery in Ambulatory and ICU Patients

Characteristics	Ambulatory	HFNC	NIV	IMV
Inhalation pathway	Oro-nasal	Nasal	Oro-nasal	Artificial airway
Aerosol carrier type	Patient inspiratory flow	Patient inspiratory flow + HFNC flow (10–60 L/min)	Patient inspiratory flow + ventilator delivery flow (30–60 L/min) and leak flow (10–30 L/min)	Patient inspiratory flow + ventilator delivery flow (30–60 L/min) or ventilator delivery flow (30–60 L/min) only
Aerosol carrier waveform	Sinusoidal	Sinusoidal + square	Sinusoidal + Descending	Sinusoidal + Descending or square or descending
Total flow	20–40 L/min	30–100 L/min	60–150 L/min	30–100 L/min
Aerosol surrounding temperature and humidity	Ambient	37 °C, 100%	31–34 °C, up to 100%	37 °C, 100%
Aerosol storage	Oro-nasal pharynx	Oro-nasal pharynx + HFNC circuit	Oro-nasal pharynx + non-vented mask	Ventilator circuit

Abbreviations: HFNC = high-flow nasal cannula; IMV = invasive mechanical ventilation; NIV = noninvasive ventilation.

hypoxemia or pulmonary hypertension, and nebulizers need to be placed in-line with respiratory support (17, 18). For other medications, placement of a nebulizer in-line with respiratory support is also commonly employed when higher than labeled doses are needed to provide relief, such as inhaled albuterol for patients with acute severe asthma (19).

FACTORS INFLUENCING OPTIMAL AEROSOL DELIVERY VIA RESPIRATORY SUPPORT DEVICES

Invasive Mechanical Ventilation

Aerosol Device

Nebulizers and pMDI with spacer could be placed in-line with an invasive mechanical ventilator. Jet nebulizers (JNs) and vibrating mesh nebulizers (VMNs) are the commonly utilized nebulizers during IMV (2, 9). JN can be operated continuously with an external gas source or intermittently with inspiration synchronized with gas flow from the ventilator. The former requires a driving gas from an external gas source, usually at a gas flow of 6–8 L/min, the introduction of the external gas flow into the ventilator system impacts ventilator settings, for example, it increases tidal volume delivery and alters the fraction of inspired oxygen (F_1O_2) to patients (9). More importantly, it interferes with the ventilator's ability to sense patient effort and makes the ventilator difficult to trigger (20). For patients with muscle weakness or severe air-trapping, the continuous JN may worsen patient-ventilator trigger asynchrony. If continuous JN is used, close monitoring of patient triggering is needed with adjustment of ventilator settings and alarms as needed and return to pre-treatment settings after completion of the nebulizer treatment. In contrast, for inspiration-synchronized JN, the driving gas flow is typically from the set volume of gas delivered to the patient. Thus, it does not affect ventilator function. Continuous aerosol causes waste during the exhalation phase; however, inspiration-synchronized nebulization does not substantially improve nebulizer efficiency and it prolongs the duration of each treatment by up to 3-fold compared to continuous operation (21).

VMNs and pMDIs are not driven by gas flow, thus, neither device affects ventilator sensors or the set ventilatory parameters. The inhaled drug dose with VMN is reported to be 2–3-fold higher than with JN (22–24) and similar to pMDI and spacer (24–26). The higher efficiency of VMNs is mainly due to a higher total output because of their low residual volume (<0.1 mL), in contrast to 0.5–1.2 mL residual volume for JNs.

Nebulizer Placement

To optimize delivery efficiency, researchers placed various nebulizers at different positions of the ventilator circuit, including between circuit and airway, in the inspiratory limb 15–80 cm from the airway, and near the ventilator (inlet and outlet of the humidifier) (22, 23, 27). With bias flow, VMN was most efficient when placed close to the ventilator (23), as bias flow carries the continuously produced aerosol into the inspiratory limb toward the patient between inspirations, resulting in a reservoir effect with a 50–80% increase in delivered dose (23). When there is no bias flow and the VMN is placed near the ventilator, a bolus of aerosol from the continuous VMN collects in the humidifier and nearby tubing, but a tidal volume of 500 mL is insufficient to carry the bolus of aerosol to the patient through the 6-foot long tubing in the inspiratory limb of the circuit (22). This explains why in the absence of bias flow the inhaled dose is higher with VMN placed close to Y-piece than at the humidifier. With a continuously operating JN, the driving gas flow carries the aerosol. In this setting, the JN output acts like the bias flow so that it is more efficient in a position closer to the humidifier without bias flow, but as bias flow is added to the circuit there is greater aerosol washout, and the inhaled dose is reduced with JN at this position.

Interestingly, when the JN is placed at the inspiratory limb close to Y-piece, the inhaled dose with the JN operated in inspiration-synchronized mode is 2–3-fold higher than that with operation in the continuous mode (28). However, when the nebulizer is placed at the inlet of the humidifier, no significant differences in the inhaled doses are found between the two modes of operation of JNs (21). Zhang et al. (27) reported that placing an inspiration-synchronized JN at a distance of 80 cm from the Y-piece in the inspiratory limb resulted in a higher inhaled dose than placing it at the inlet of the humidifier or between the endotracheal tube and Y-piece. However, the inspiratory limb of the ventilator heated wire circuit is usually 150–160 cm long and disconnecting such circuits to place an aerosol device is not feasible.

Reservoir Volume and Placement for pMDI

pMDIs cannot be directly placed in-line with the ventilator circuit, they are connected via a reservoir device or adapter with two open ports (Figure 11.3). The inhaled dose is significantly lower with a reservoir volume less than 150 mL than that with a reservoir volume higher than 150 mL (24, 26, 29). The pMDI and the reservoir chamber need to be placed at the Y-piece of the inspiratory limb. Notably, with an adapter that has a very small volume (20–30 mL), the aerosol efficiency was found to be low at regular tidal volume settings (29). With adapters that had a 90-degree right-angled bend, aerosol delivery was even lower (26).

Humidification

During invasive ventilation, administration of dry gases may irritate the airway, and cause dryness of the airway mucosa leading to mucociliary dysfunction, mucus plugging, and atelectasis. Accordingly, providing heat and humidification of the inspired gases is essential in a patient with an artificial airway (30). Active humidifiers heat the water in the chamber, which heats and humidifies dry air when it passes over the chamber. In contrast, passive humidifiers, called heat-moisture exchangers (HMEs), are placed between the ventilator circuit and the airway to capture heat and humidity from exhaled gases, which are in turn used to heat and humidify the inhaled gases. As most HMEs filter aerosol particles, they must be removed or bypassed during aerosol delivery. Alternatively, the nebulizer can be placed between the HME and patient, but exhaled aerosols can build up on the HME and increase the resistance to airflow imparted by the HME over time.

Most medical aerosols are hygroscopic and grow larger when passing into the gas with high absolute humidity. This can occur in a heated ventilator circuit, or as inhaled aerosol encounters the exhaled heat and humidity in the airway. Consequently, the inhaled dose is reduced by ~50% in heated circuits compared to dry circuits (22, 31, 32). However, turning off the active heater to deliver aerosol within 10 minutes does not improve aerosol delivery efficiency (33), as the circuits are not completely dry and cooled down in this short interval. Interestingly, when using models which exhale heat and humidity, the placement of an aerosol device near the patient shows little to no change in delivery efficiency with the dry vs wet circuits (34). As such, it is not recommended to turn off the active heater for the sole purpose of improving aerosol delivery. For antibiotics or other cost-prohibitive medications, considering that it may take a long period for a humidifier and circuits to cool down, using an HME rather than an active heater for humidification might be a practical solution; nebulizers can bypass the HME or be placed between the HME and the patient (35).

In summary, the use of VMN or pMDI with a spacer is preferred for optimal aerosol delivery in patients with chronic obstructive pulmonary disease (COPD) and asthma during invasive ventilation and a JN is a less efficient alternative. When a VMN is utilized, it is recommended to place the VMN at the inlet of the humidifier in the presence of bias flow, or in the inspiratory limb close to the Y-piece in the absence of bias flow in the circuit. When a pMDI is utilized, a spacer with a minimum volume of 150 mL placed in the inspiratory limb close to the Y-piece is recommended. If an HME is used, it must be removed or bypassed during aerosol delivery. If the patient uses an active heater for humidification, it is not recommended to turn off the heater for routine aerosol therapy.

Evaluation of Treatment Effects

The inhaled dose during invasive ventilation varies, due to patient characteristics such as the severity of airway obstruction, lung function, breathing efforts, etc., and the aforementioned factors influencing aerosol delivery (Figure 11.1). Assessment of treatment effects could help to titrate the nominal dose for individual patients. For example, when a bronchodilator is utilized, the bronchodilator responses can be assessed via the changes in the airway resistance and intrinsic positive end-expiratory pressure (PEEPi) for patients with COPD and asthma (13). For other inhaled medications such as corticosteroids or antibiotics, which do not generate immediate airway responses, the measurement of bronchoalveolar lavage or systemic levels can help to provide guidance regarding the optimal drug dose (36). In patients receiving mechanical ventilation, the upper airway is bypassed by an artificial airway so that the systemic levels of the aerosolized medication reflect the dose deposited in the lower airway. Thus, the concentrations of the aerosolized medication in the urine or blood could be used to evaluate the aerosol delivery efficiency and serve as guides to determine the appropriate nominal dose.

Tracheostomy/laryngectomy Patients without Invasive Mechanical Ventilation

Clinically, some patients in the ICU may not require ventilator support but still need to maintain an open airway, such as a tracheostomy. When they require aerosol therapy, although their upper airway is intact, using conventional aerosol therapy with a mask or mouthpiece has low aerosol delivery efficiency (37), as most of the tidal volume is delivered via the tracheostomy rather than the upper airway. Additionally, the tracheostomy tube creates a barrier for aerosol inhalation via the upper airway. If the patients have a cuffed tracheostomy tube or have undergone a laryngectomy, which completely bypasses the upper airway, patients could only breathe in and out via the tracheostomy or laryngectomy. In such patients, aerosol delivery is achieved via tracheostomy or laryngectomy (Figure 11.4).

In patients with a tracheostomy collar, JN can be used via an extension tubing to maintain the nebulizer cup in a vertical position (Figure 11.4a) or with a T-piece (Figure 11.4b). For patients requiring humidification, JN or VMN can be placed in-line with the humidification circuit (Figure 11.4c and d) without interrupting humidification. Notably, placing the nebulizer close to the patient (Figure 11.4e and f) in the humidification setup generated a lower inhaled dose than directly placing the nebulizer with an extension tubing (Figure 11.4a and b) (34). When a pMDI is used, an open-ended spacer is needed to connect the pMDI

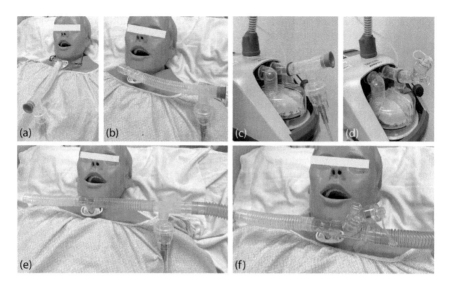

Figure 11.4 Schematic showing nebulizer setups for patients with a tracheostomy demonstrated on a mannikin. A jet nebulizer is connected to a tracheostomy collar via an extension tubing (panel a) or via a T-piece (panel b), with the other end capped. When heated humidification is provided, a jet nebulizer (panel c) or a vibrating mesh nebulizer (panel d) is placed at the humidifier. When cool aerosol is provided via T-piece, a jet nebulizer (panel e) or a vibrating mesh nebulizer (panel f) is placed close to the T-piece.

with the tracheostomy or laryngectomy tube (Figure 11.3). A pMDI should be actuated at the beginning of inspiration, and patients are allowed to breathe in and out via the spacer several times. A manual resuscitator connected with the spacer has been employed to deliver breaths for patients during aerosol delivery. However, an in vitro study found that the inhaled mass with the assistance of manual ventilation was similar to that achieved with spontaneous breathing via various aerosol devices that were placed in-line with the tracheostomy (38).

Non-invasive Ventilation

Unlike IMV, NIV uses a mask or helmet rather than an endotracheal or tracheostomy tube to access the airway. As masks tend to leak, compensation for changing levels of leaks is required, implying that gas flows are higher and more turbulent than those during IMV (Table 11.3). Two types of ventilators are employed for NIV. A single-limb bi-level ventilator driven by a turbine is most commonly utilized, and this ventilator adjusts flow through a fixed orifice exhalation valve placed between the circuit and mask to compensate for the mask leak. More recently, dual-limb conventional critical care ventilators have been equipped with modules to provide NIV.

Aerosol Device Type and Placement

Only continuous JN, VMN, or pMDI with spacer could be placed in-line with single-limb ventilators to deliver aerosolized medication (Figures 11.2 and 11.5). Due to the negligible residual volume, VMNs have a higher delivery efficiency than JNs (39, 40). Aerosol devices placed between the mask and the exhalation valve provide higher aerosol delivery efficiency than placement close to the ventilator

(41–43). Placing the aerosol device closer to the ventilator allows the aerosol to be flushed through and leak from the exhalation valve, while placing the aerosol device between the mask and the exhalation valve reduces such losses. The addition of a 15 cm extension tubing between the VMN and the exhalation valve further enhances aerosol delivery (41), due to the reservoir effect of the extension tubing. However, the added volume of the tubing could increase the dead space, which may be detrimental for patients with asthma or COPD. When dual-limb ventilators are used for NIV, there is no fixed leak in the circuit but air leaks from face masks continue to be a factor in reducing the efficiency of aerosol delivery.

NIV Interface

NIV can be connected to patients via a nasal mask, a full face mask, a total face mask, or a helmet. Full face masks are the most commonly used interfaces and two types are commonly employed: vented masks with the exhalation port incorporated (only used with a single-limb circuit) or non-vented masks. The use of vented masks greatly reduces aerosol delivery efficiency (42, 43) and they are not recommended. Only non-vented masks should be employed during aerosol delivery via NIV.

Ventilator Type

VMNs placed in optimal positions in the single-limb ventilator and dual-limb ventilator achieve similar efficacy of inhaled dose delivery (43). The optimal position in a single-limb circuit is 15 cm away from the exhalation valve and close to the mask, whereas in a dual-limb circuit placement of the VMN is optimal in the inspiratory limb at a distance of 15 cm from the Y-piece.

Humidification

In contrast to IMV, turning off humidification during aerosol delivery via NIV does not improve aerosol delivery (44), probably because NIV employs gases with a lower temperature and absolute humidity than IMV.

In summary, to optimize aerosol delivery via NIV, the use of a VMN or a pMDI with a spacer provides more efficient aerosol delivery than a JN. Aerosol devices should be placed between the non-vented mask and the exhalation valve in the single-limb ventilator or 15 cm away from the Y-piece in the inspiratory limb of the dual-limb ventilator. A pMDI should be actuated at the beginning of inspiration. Vented masks should be avoided during aerosol delivery. Turning off the humidifier does not improve aerosol delivery during NIV.

High-flow Nasal Cannula

High-flow nasal cannula provides heated and humidified gas for patients, with the gas flow set higher than the patient's peak inspiratory flow during tidal breathing. Oxygen therapy with HFNC is now being increasingly utilized for patients with COPD because high-flow gas washes out the dead space in the upper airway, thereby reducing $PaCO_2$ and the work of breathing (45). HFNC is an ideal platform to continuously deliver aerosolized medication to patients (46). Unlike NIV, HFNC can be used continuously for days, even weeks, as the probability of skin breakdown or discomfort from the continuous use of HFNC is much lower than that with a tightly fitted mask. Moreover, HFNC flows are lower and more laminar than flows employed during NIV (**Table 11.3**).

Transnasal pulmonary aerosol delivery via HFNC has become popular in ICUs worldwide and key factors influencing the efficiency of drug delivery have been explored in multiple in vitro and in vivo studies (5, 47–51). Notably, aerosol administration with JN and a mask or mouthpiece while HFNC is in use decreases the inhaled dose compared to aerosol administered through the

HFNC (47), thus, the concurrent use of a nebulizer with a mask/mouthpiece during HFNC treatment should be avoided (11).

Nebulizer Types

During aerosol administration via HFNC, VMNs deliver several-fold higher drug doses than JNs (48, 49). Additionally, JNs require external-driven gas (usual gas flow of 6–8 L/min), which limits their use in patients who need HFNC gas flow less than 8 L/min, such as in small children. The use of JN in-line with HFNC alters the gas flow, humidity, and F_1O_2, which might cause malfunction for some HFNC devices, such as Airvo2 (Fisher & Paykel, Auckland, New Zealand). In contrast, VMNs are preferred for aerosol delivery via HFNC because they are driven by electricity and no external gas flow is needed for their operation.

Nebulizer Placement

In adults and older children, the inhaled drug dose is higher with the nebulizer placed at the humidifier than when it is placed close to the nasal cannula, especially at low flow settings (49–51). Aerosol particles leaving the nasal prongs are <2.1 µm in diameter, as larger particles generated by aerosol devices rain out either in the humidifier, circuit, or nasal prongs where the condensation can occlude gas flow. More of the aerosol emitted by a VMN placed before or after the humidifier chamber during exhalation is available to be inhaled in the next inspiration, reducing the waste of aerosol. In contrast, nebulizer placement close to the cannula has a more limited reservoir for collecting aerosol between inspirations.

Gas Flow Settings

By definition, HFNC gas flows are typically set to meet or exceed a patient's tidal peak inspiratory flow, so as to reduce air entrainment and also generate a certain level of positive airway pressure (52). Unfortunately, gas flow higher than a patient's tidal peak inspiratory flow during aerosol administration reduces inhaled drug dose by increasing waste of aerosol. With medium gas flows (15–30 L/min for adults and 0.5–1.0 L/min/kg for young children), in vitro models report higher inhaled drug dose with distressed breathing than with quiet relaxed breathing (49–51, 53, 54). Setting the HFNC gas flow lower than the patient's tidal peak inspiratory flow benefits transnasal aerosol delivery. In fact, HFNC flow set at 50% of the patient's tidal peak inspiratory flow was shown to be more comfortable and to provide higher pulmonary drug delivery compared to higher HFNC flows (55, 56).

Tidal peak inspiratory flow varies in different patients and there is no commercially available device to provide a breath-by-breath measurement of patient's tidal peak inspiratory flow. Most adult patients with acute respiratory failure do not spontaneously generate peak flows above 40 L/min during tidal breathing (52). For patients with acute hypoxemic respiratory failure, a pragmatic solution is to titrate down gas flow with high F_1O_2 to provide acceptable target oxygen saturations prior to aerosol administration. Empirically titrating the HFNC flow down to 20–25 L/min for adult patients with acute respiratory failure or 15–20 L/min for adult patients who are not in acute respiratory distress, or 0.5 L/min/kg for young children could provide efficient aerosol delivery with HFNC (11).

Assessment of patient responses to inhaled medication, such as improvement of oxygenation or pulmonary arterial pressure for inhaled epoprostenol (17), or the increment of forced expiratory volume in one second (FEV_1) for inhaled albuterol can provide confidence on appropriate dosing (56, 57). Notably, when the flow is titrated down during aerosol delivery, HFNC benefits such as constant F_IO_2 or reduction of work of breathing would be compromised, thus closely monitoring the patient responses is warranted. If needed, a concentrated drug solution could be used to shorten the duration of low flow settings for aerosol delivery (58).

In summary, a VMN placed at the inlet of the humidifier is preferred for aerosol delivery via HFNC. HFNC gas flows need to be titrated down to a tolerable low flow during aerosol delivery for optimal nebulizer efficiency.

FUGITIVE AEROSOLS AND MITIGATION STRATEGIES

Nebulizers generate a significant amount of fugitive aerosols, even for patients who do not have airborne diseases. Reducing the second-hand inhalation of fugitive aerosols would be beneficial for healthcare workers. Invasive ventilation is a closed system and filters should be placed at the outlet of the ventilator, whether or not aerosol is being administered. During nebulization, the fugitive aerosols leaked from the invasive ventilator would be minimal, depending on the type of filter used. Placing a filter at the expiratory port of the ventilator reduces fugitive aerosols and also protects the expiratory flow sensor (35). Notably, the filter may become obstructed with aerosols over time, increasing the expiratory resistance, thus it needs to be frequently changed especially during continuous nebulization. For NIV, when a nebulizer is placed between the mask and the exhalation port in the single-limb ventilator, a filter needs to be placed between the nebulizer and exhalation valve (Figure 11.5) or at the exhalation port (59). For HFNC, placing a procedure mask over the patient's face reduces fugitive aerosols, with and without medical aerosol administration (60).

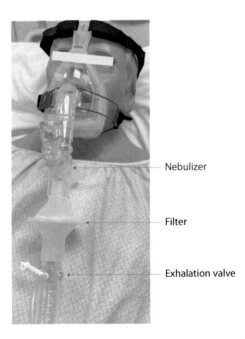

Nebulizer

Filter

Exhalation valve

Figure 11.5 During noninvasive ventilation using a single-limb circuit, a vibrating mesh nebulizer is placed between the exhalation valve and the mask. A filter is placed between the nebulizer and the exhalation valve to reduce the release of fugitive aerosols into the room environment.

147

CONCLUSION

Compared to ambulatory patients, aerosol therapy for patients in the ICU needing respiratory support is challenging, due to a host of factors influencing drug delivery. In addition to patient characteristics and the features of the aerosol generators, the configuration of the respiratory support devices, such as device settings, placement of the aerosol generator, and humidification, influence aerosol delivery, resulting in variable inhaled doses. Understanding these factors can help to optimize aerosol delivery for patients in the ICU. Close monitoring of patient responses and adjustment of respiratory support device settings and nominal doses are also necessary. With careful attention to techniques of administration, aerosolized therapies are effective for patients in the ICU.

REFERENCES

1. Society of Critical Care Medicine (SCCM). SCCM | Critical Care Statistics. [cited 2022 July 19]. Available from: https://sccm.org/Communications/Critical-Care-Statistics
2. Reva Research Network, AT@ICU Study Group, Ehrmann S, et al. Aerosol therapy in intensive and intermediate care units: Prospective observation of 2808 critically ill patients. Intensive Care Med 2016;42(2):192–201. DOI:10.1007/s00134-015-4114-5
3. Lyu S, Li J, Wu M, et al. The use of aerosolized medications in adult intensive care unit patients: A prospective, multicenter, observational, cohort study. J Aerosol Med Pulm Drug Deliv 2021;34(6):383–391. DOI:10.1089/jamp.2021.0004
4. Lyu S, Li J, Yang L, et al. The utilization of aerosol therapy in mechanical ventilation patients: A prospective multicenter observational cohort study and a review of the current evidence. Ann Transl Med 2020;8(17):14.
5. Li J, Tu M, Yang L, et al. Worldwide clinical practice of high-flow nasal cannula and concomitant aerosol therapy in the adult ICU setting. Respir Care 2021;66(9):1416–1424. DOI:10.4187/respcare.08996
6. MacIntyre NR, Silver RM, Miller CW, et al. Aerosol delivery in intubated, mechanically ventilated patients. Crit Care Med 1985;13(2):81–84. DOI:10.1097/00003246-198502000-00005
7. Wong FJ, Dudney T, Dhand R. Aerosolized antibiotics for treatment of pneumonia in mechanically ventilated subjects. Respir Care 2019;64(8): 962–979. DOI:10.4187/respcare.07024
8. Dhand R. Inhalation therapy in invasive and noninvasive mechanical ventilation. Curr Opin Crit Care 2007;13(1):27–38. DOI:10.1097/MCC.0b013e328012e022
9. Dugernier J, Ehrmann S, Sottiaux T, et al. Aerosol delivery during invasive mechanical ventilation: A systematic review. Crit Care 2017;21(1):264. DOI:10.1186/s13054-017-1844-5
10. Dhand R. Aerosol therapy in patients receiving noninvasive positive pressure ventilation. J Aerosol Med Pulm Drug Deliv 2012;25(2):63–78. DOI:10.1089/jamp.2011.0929
11. Li J, Fink JB, MacLoughlin R, et al. A narrative review on trans-nasal pulmonary aerosol delivery. Crit Care 2020;24(1):506. DOI:10.1186/s13054-020-03206-9
12. Dhand R, Tobin MJ. Bronchodilator delivery with metered-dose inhalers in mechanically-ventilated patients. Eur Respir J 1996;9(3):585–595. DOI:10.1183/09031936.96.09030585

13. Dhand R, Tobin MJ. Inhaled bronchodilator therapy in mechanically ventilated patients. Am J Respir Crit Care Med 1997;156(1):3–10. DOI:10.1164/ajrccm.156.1.9610025

14. Pleasants RA, Hess DR. Aerosol delivery devices for obstructive lung diseases. Respir Care 2018;63(6):708–733. DOI:10.4187/respcare.06290

15. Diot P, Morra L, Smaldone GC. Albuterol delivery in a model of mechanical ventilation. Comparison of metered-dose inhaler and nebulizer efficiency. Am J Respir Crit Care Med 1995;152(4 Pt 1):1391–1394. DOI:10.1164/ajrccm.152.4.7551401

16. Dhand R. Inhalation therapy with metered-dose inhalers and dry powder inhalers in mechanically ventilated patients. Respir Care 2005;50(10): 1331–1334; discussion 1344–1345.

17. Li J, Gurnani PK, Roberts KM, et al. The clinical impact of flow titration on epoprostenol delivery via high flow nasal cannula for ICU patients with pulmonary hypertension or right ventricular dysfunction: A retrospective cohort comparison study. J Clin Med 2020;9(2):464. DOI:10.3390/jcm9020464

18. Chen SH, Chen LK, Teng TH, et al. Comparison of inhaled nitric oxide with aerosolized prostacyclin or analogues for the postoperative management of pulmonary hypertension: A systematic review and meta-analysis. Ann Med 2020;52(3–4):120–130. DOI:10.1080/07853890.2020.1746826

19. Rodrigo GJ, Rodrigo C. Continuous vs intermittent beta-agonists in the treatment of acute adult asthma: A systematic review with meta-analysis. Chest 2002;122(1):160–165. DOI:10.1378/chest.122.1.160

20. Beaty CD, Ritz RH, Benson MS. Continuous in-line nebulizers complicate pressure support ventilation. Chest 1989;96(6):1360–1363. DOI:10.1378/chest.96.6.1360

21. Wan GH, Lin HL, Fink JB, et al. In vitro evaluation of aerosol delivery by different nebulization modes in pediatric and adult mechanical ventilators. Respir Care 2014;59(10):1494–1500. DOI:10.4187/respcare.02999

22. Ari A, Areabi H, Fink JB. Evaluation of aerosol generator devices at 3 locations in humidified and non-humidified circuits during adult mechanical ventilation. Respir Care 2010;55(7):837–844.

23. Ari A, Atalay OT, Harwood R, et al. Influence of nebulizer type, position, and bias flow on aerosol drug delivery in simulated pediatric and adult lung models during mechanical ventilation. Respir Care 2010;55(7):845–851.

24. Naughton PJ, Joyce M, Mac Giolla Eain M, et al. Evaluation of aerosol drug delivery options during adult mechanical ventilation in the COVID-19 era. Pharmaceutics 2021;13(10):1574. DOI:10.3390/pharmaceutics13101574

25. Ari A, Harwood RJ, Sheard MM, et al. Pressurized metered-dose inhalers versus nebulizers in the treatment of mechanically ventilated subjects with artificial airways: An in vitro study. Respir Care 2015;60(11):1570–1574. DOI:10.4187/respcare.04125

26. Marik P, Hogan J, Krikorian J. A comparison of bronchodilator therapy delivered by nebulization and metered-dose inhaler in mechanically ventilated patients. Chest 1999;115(6):1653–1657. DOI:10.1378/chest.115.6.1653

27. Zhang C, Mi J, Zhang Z, et al. The clinical practice and best aerosol delivery location in intubated and mechanically ventilated patients: A randomized clinical trial. Biomed Res Int 2021;2021:6671671. DOI:10.1155/2021/6671671

28. Miller DD, Amin MM, Palmer LB, et al. Aerosol delivery and modern mechanical ventilation: In vitro/in vivo evaluation. Am J Respir Crit Care Med 2003;168(10):1205–1209. DOI:10.1164/rccm.200210-1167OC

29. Boukhettala N, Porée T, Diot P, et al. In vitro performance of spacers for aerosol delivery during adult mechanical ventilation. J Aerosol Med Pulm Drug Deliv 2015;28(2):130–136. DOI:10.1089/jamp.2013.1091

30. American Association for Respiratory Care, Restrepo RD, Walsh BK. Humidification during invasive and noninvasive mechanical ventilation: 2012. Respir Care 2012;57(5):782–788. DOI:10.4187/respcare.01766

31. Fink JB, Dhand R, Grychowski J, et al. Reconciling in vitro and in vivo measurements of aerosol delivery from a metered-dose inhaler during mechanical ventilation and defining efficiency-enhancing factors. Am J Respir Crit Care Med 1999;159(1):63–68. DOI:10.1164/ajrccm.159.1.9803119

32. Fink JB, Dhand R, Duarte AG, et al. Aerosol delivery from a metered-dose inhaler during mechanical ventilation. An in vitro model. Am J Respir Crit Care Med 1996;154(2 Pt 1):382–387. DOI:10.1164/ajrccm.154.2.8756810

33. Lin HL, Fink JB, Zhou Y, et al. Influence of moisture accumulation in inline spacer on delivery of aerosol using metered-dose inhaler during mechanical ventilation. Respir Care 2009;54(10):1336–1341.

34. Ari A, Harwood R, Sheard M, et al. Quantifying aerosol delivery in simulated spontaneously breathing patients with tracheostomy using different humidification systems with or without exhaled humidity. Respir Care 2016;61(5):600–606. DOI:10.4187/respcare.04127

35. Rello J, Rouby JJ, Sole-Lleonart C, et al. Key considerations on nebulization of antimicrobial agents to mechanically ventilated patients. Clin Microbiol Infect 2017;23(9):640–646. DOI:10.1016/j.cmi.2017.03.018

36. Luyt CE, Eldon MA, Stass H, et al. Pharmacokinetics and tolerability of amikacin administered as BAY41-6551 aerosol in mechanically ventilated patients with Gram-negative pneumonia and acute renal failure. J Aerosol Med Pulm Drug Deliv 2011;24(4):183–190. DOI:10.1089/jamp.2010.0860

37. Bugis AA, Sheard MM, Fink JB, et al. Comparison of aerosol delivery by face mask and tracheostomy collar. Respir Care 2015;60(9):1220–1226.

38. Alhamad BR, Fink JB, Harwood RJ, et al. Effect of aerosol devices and administration techniques on drug delivery in a simulated spontaneously breathing pediatric tracheostomy model. Respir Care 2015;60(7):1026–1032.

39. Galindo-Filho VC, Ramos ME, Rattes CSF, et al. Radioaerosol pulmonary deposition using mesh and jet nebulizers during noninvasive ventilation in healthy subjects. Respir Care 2015;60(9):1238–1246. DOI:10.4187/respcare.03667

40. Galindo-Filho VC, Alcoforado L, Rattes C, et al. A mesh nebulizer is more effective than jet nebulizer to nebulize bronchodilators during noninvasive ventilation of subjects with COPD: A randomized controlled trial with radiolabeled aerosols. Respir Med 2019;153:60–67. DOI:10.1016/j.rmed.2019.05.016

41. Michotte JB, Jossen E, Roeseler J, et al. In vitro comparison of five nebulizers during noninvasive ventilation: Analysis of inhaled and lost doses. J Aerosol Med Pulm Drug Deliv 2014;27(6):430–440. DOI:10.1089/jamp.2013.1070

42. Tan W, Dai B, Lu CL, et al. The effect of different interfaces on the aerosol delivery with vibrating mesh nebulizer during noninvasive positive pressure ventilation. J Aerosol Med Pulm Drug Deliv 2021;34(6):366–373. DOI:10.1089/jamp.2020.1623

43. Tan W, Dai B, Xu DY, et al. In-vitro comparison of single limb and dual limb circuit for aerosol delivery via noninvasive ventilation. Respir Care 2022;67(7):807–813.
44. Saeed H, Elberry AA, Eldin AS, et al. Effect of nebulizer designs on aerosol delivery during non-invasive mechanical ventilation: A modeling study of in vitro data. Pulm Ther 2017;3(1):233–241. DOI:10.1007/s41030-017-0033-7
45. Huang X, Du Y, Ma Z, et al. High-flow nasal cannula oxygen versus conventional oxygen for hypercapnic chronic obstructive pulmonary disease: A meta-analysis of randomized controlled trials. Clin Respir J 2021;15(4):437–444. DOI:10.1111/crj.13317
46. Levy SD, Alladina JW, Hibbert KA, et al. High-flow oxygen therapy and other inhaled therapies in intensive care units. Lancet 2016;387(10030): 1867–1878. DOI:10.1016/S0140-6736(16)30245-8
47. Bennett G, Joyce M, Fernández EF, et al. Comparison of aerosol delivery across combinations of drug delivery interfaces with and without concurrent high-flow nasal therapy. Intensive Care Med Exp 2019;7(1):20. DOI:10.1186/s40635-019-0245-2
48. Dugernier J, Hesse M, Jumetz T, et al. Aerosol delivery with two nebulizers through high-flow nasal cannula: A randomized cross-over single-photon emission computed tomography-computed tomography study. J Aerosol Med Pulm Drug Deliv 2017;30(5):349–358. DOI:10.1089/jamp.2017.1366
49. Li J, Williams L, Fink JB. The impact of high-flow nasal cannula device, nebulizer type, and placement on trans-nasal aerosol drug delivery. Respir Care 2022;67(1):1–8. DOI:10.4187/respcare.09133
50. Li J, Wu W, Fink JB. In vitro comparison between inspiration synchronized and continuous vibrating mesh nebulizer during trans-nasal aerosol delivery. Intensive Care Med Exp 2020;8(1):6. DOI:10.1186/s40635-020-0293-7
51. Li J, Gong L, Ari A, et al. Decrease the flow setting to improve trans-nasal pulmonary aerosol delivery via "high-flow nasal cannula" to infants and toddlers. Pediatr Pulmonol 2019;54(6):914–921. DOI:10.1002/ppul.24274
52. Li J, Scott JB, Fink JB, et al. Optimizing high-flow nasal cannula flow settings in adult hypoxemic patients based on peak inspiratory flow during tidal breathing. Ann Intensive Care 2021;11(1):164. DOI:10.1186/s13613-021-00949-8
53. Réminiac F, Vecellio L, Heuzé-Vourc'h N, et al. Aerosol therapy in adults receiving high flow nasal cannula oxygen therapy. J Aerosol Med Pulm Drug Deliv 2016;29(2):134–141. DOI:10.1089/jamp.2015.1219
54. Dailey PA, Harwood R, Walsh K, et al. Aerosol delivery through adult high flow nasal cannula with heliox and oxygen. Respir Care 2017;62(9): 1186–1192. DOI:10.4187/respcare.05127
55. Li J, Gong L, Fink JB. The ratio of nasal cannula gas flow to patient inspiratory flow on trans-nasal pulmonary aerosol delivery for adults: An in vitro study. Pharmaceutics 2019;11(5):225. DOI:10.3390/pharmaceutics11050225
56. Li J, Chen Y, Ehrmann S, et al. Bronchodilator delivery via high-flow nasal cannula: A randomized controlled trial to compare the effects of gas flows. Pharmaceutics 2021;13(10):1655. DOI:10.3390/pharmaceutics13101655
57. Li J, Zhao M, Hadeer M, et al. Dose response to transnasal pulmonary administration of bronchodilator aerosols via nasal high-flow therapy in adults with stable chronic obstructive pulmonary disease and asthma. Respiration 2019;98(5):401–409. DOI:10.1159/000501564

58. Li J, Wu W, Fink JB. In vitro comparison of unit dose vs infusion pump administration of albuterol via high-flow nasal cannula in toddlers. Pediatr Pulmonol 2020;55(2):322–329. DOI:10.1002/ppul.24589

59. Kaur R, Weiss TT, Perez A, et al. Practical strategies to reduce nosocomial transmission to healthcare professionals providing respiratory care to patients with COVID-19. Crit Care 2020;24(1):571. DOI:10.1186/s13054-020-03231-8

60. Li J, Alolaiwat AA, Harnois LJ, et al. Mitigating fugitive aerosols during aerosol delivery via high-flow nasal cannula devices. Respir Care 2022;67(4):404–414. DOI:10.4187/respcare.09589

12 Inhaled Therapy for Other Respiratory Diseases

Cystic Fibrosis and Non-Cystic Fibrosis Bronchiectasis

Mahmoud Ibrahim, MD and Alexander G. Duarte, MD

CONTENTS

INTRODUCTION

Once regarded as an orphan disease, bronchiectasis is now recognized more frequently due to greater clinician awareness, increased chest tomography (CT) availability, and genetic testing (1). Bronchiectasis may be classified as related to cystic fibrosis (CF) or non-cystic fibrosis. Bronchiectasis related to CF arises from genetic mutations in the cystic fibrosis transmembrane conductance regulator (CFTR) gene that give rise to defective airway epithelial ion transport and altered mucociliary clearance. In contrast, non-CF bronchiectasis (NCFB) represents a diverse set of conditions associated with altered mucociliary clearance, airway inflammation, and airway infections not associated with CFTR gene mutations.

In management of CF and NCFB, inhalation therapy is a preferred method of drug delivery as medication that directly deposits on the airway provides therapeutic benefits with reduced systemic side effects. Therapies to prevent, relieve, and treat airway narrowing, secretion accumulation, inflammation, and microbial infections associated with bronchiectasis include bronchodilators, corticosteroids, mucolytics, and antimicrobials. Moreover, many professional society guidelines recommend various inhalation therapies as a prominent form of drug administration in patients with bronchiectasis (2, 3).

BRONCHODILATORS

Bronchodilators are frequently prescribed for dyspnea relief and the US Bronchiectasis Research Registry found that 61% of patients with non-CF bronchiectasis were prescribed a bronchodilator (4). Yet, evidence-based data to indicate that bronchodilators are effective at a population level are lacking. A systematic review examined the effectiveness of short-acting β-agonists or anticholinergics in children and adults with bronchiectasis were unable to identify adequately designed trials (5). Evidence to support the use of long-acting bronchodilators to improve lung function, mucociliary clearance, or dyspnea relief in patients with bronchiectasis is even less robust (6). For the individual patient, short-acting β-agonists and/or short-acting antimuscarinics may provide dyspnea relief and aid in the clearance of secretions. They may also mitigate excessive coughing associated with mucolytic therapy-associated bronchospasm (7). As for the delivery device, preference should be guided by convenience, ease of administration, and availability. Pressurized metered dose inhaler (pMDI) delivery of short-acting β-agonists or soft mist inhaler delivery of combined short-acting β-agonists and/or short-acting antimuscarinics is acceptable. Jet nebulizer delivery of short-acting bronchodilators is a common method that may be more convenient for a given patient but additional research is needed to assess clinical efficacy, patient preference, and outcomes with nebulizer delivery using adaptive aerosol delivery or vibrating mesh technology (8).

CORTICOSTEROIDS

As bronchiectasis is associated with neutrophilic airway inflammation, clinicians may feel compelled to prescribe inhaled corticosteroids, although this therapy is primarily effective in eosinophilic airway disease. However, inhaled corticosteroids are prescribed to 44% of patients with CF and 39% of patients with non-CF bronchiectasis (4, 9). Yet, a US consensus group that examined findings from 8 clinical trials involving 419 subjects with CF did not find supporting evidence of benefits from the use of inhaled corticosteroids regarding lung function, quality of life, and exacerbation rates (10). Similarly, the European Society of CF recommendations indicates that inhaled corticosteroids have no proven efficacy, outside of the treatment of concomitant asthma (11). For adults with NCFB, a review of the short-term effects of inhaled corticosteroid administration found no improvement in pulmonary function tests, exacerbations rates, or health-related outcomes (2, 12). Studies included inhaled corticosteroids delivered via pMDI (13, 14). Of note, concerns about inhaled corticosteroids increasing airway bacterial density and association with an increased risk for pneumonia and nontuberculous mycobacterial (NTM) lung infections limit their use in bronchiectasis (15, 16). In summary, the risks seem to outweigh the benefits of inhaled corticosteroid use in patients with bronchiectasis.

MUCOLYTICS

In patients with bronchiectasis, mucus hyperconcentration and airway mucus stasis result in ciliary dysfunction that contribute to airway inflammation and lung infections. Consequently, therapeutic agents that decrease mucus concentration through rehydration of airway surface liquid can decrease mucus viscosity and facilitate clearance of secretions. In patients with CF, hypertonic saline reduces IL-8 levels in sputum and bronchoalveolar lavage fluid, consistent with an anti-inflammatory effect (9). Moreover, hypertonic saline administration via Pari LC plus jet nebulizer to children and adults with CF over 48 weeks yielded significant improvements in lung function and reduced exacerbations (17). A Cochrane review found improved outcomes in patients receiving inhaled hypertonic saline (7%) compared to control subjects (18). In patients with NCFB, administration of jet nebulized 7% saline over 3 months improved lung function and health-related quality of life and decreased antibiotic use compared to nebulized saline (0.9%) (19). The comparison of 6% and 0.9% saline administration by mesh nebulizer to 40 subjects with NCFB over 12 months yielded improved lung function and quality of life (20). Thus, nebulized saline is a safe and effective mucolytic agent, but the optimal solution tonicity and type of nebulizer that are needed for optimal efficacy in NCFB require further investigation.

Administration of dry powder mannitol (Pharmaxis, Sydney, Australia) by Orbital delivery device to rehydrate the airways of patients with CF revealed improvements in lung function (21, 22). Dry powder inhaled mannitol (400 mg twice daily) is approved for use in adults with CF, as an add-on therapy to standard practice, in the EU, UK, and Australia. In 2020, dry powder mannitol received FDA approval as an add-on maintenance therapy for adults with CF (23). In contrast, in patients with NCFB, a 52-week international trial assessed dry powder mannitol in 461 subjects and found no significant difference in exacerbation rates between the study and control groups (23). In addition, a systematic review of patients with NCFB found no significant improvements in lung function, quality of life, exacerbation rates, and health care utilization with mannitol administered as a dry powder inhaler (24, 25). Another class of mucolytics is N-acetylcysteine and other thiol derivatives that break disulfide bonds leading to reduced mucus viscosity. A Cochrane Review identified clinical trials of nebulized thiol derivatives and, while they were generally well tolerated, no significant benefit was observed in patients with CF (26).

Dornase alfa (Pulmozyme, Genentech, San Francisco, CA, USA) is a purified solution of the recombinant enzyme, human DNase, which reduces mucus viscosity by cleaving airway extracellular DNA released from neutrophils. A systematic review examined 19 trials involving infants to adults with CF and the authors reported improvements in lung function and reduced exacerbation rates (27). For effective lower airway deposition, dornase alfa is administered via regulatory agency-approved devices including Pari eRapid (vibrating mesh) and jet nebulizer and compressor systems; Pari-Proneb, Pari Baby, Pulmo-Aide, Mobilaire, and Porta-Neb (9). In contrast, nebulized dornase alfa has not been shown to be effective in patients with NCFB. A multicenter study compared twice daily dornase alfa and placebo over 6 months in 349 adults with NCFB and found that the use of dornase alfa was associated with more frequent exacerbations and a greater decline in FEV_1 (28). Thus, while there are clinical similarities among patients with bronchiectasis, extrapolation of clinical trial data from the CF population to the non-CF population is not recommended.

ANTIBIOTICS

Since 1945, several antibiotics have been administered by inhalation for the treatment of chronic airway infections (Table 12.1) (29). In the last decade of the

Table 12.1: Approved Antibiotic Formulation and Delivery Devices

Drug	Brand Name	Manufacturer	Formulation	Device
Aztreonam	Cayston	Gilead	Solution	Mesh nebulizer
Colistin	Colobreathe	Forest Labs	Powder	Turbospin
Colistin	ColoMycin	Xellia	Solution	Jet and mesh nebulizer
Tobramycin	TOBI	Novartis	Solution	Jet nebulizer
Tobramycin	TOBI	Novartis	Powder	T-326 inhaler
Tobramycin	Bramitob/Bethkis Tobramycin USP	Chiesi, Teva	Solution	Jet nebulizer

Table 12.2: Inhaled Antibiotics for the Treatment of Cystic Fibrosis Bronchiectasis

Author & Publication Year	Drug Dose & Frequency	Delivery Device	Subjects (N)	Primary Outcomes	Results
Ramsey, 1999	Tobramycin 300 mg bid Administered on 28-day cycle	PARI LC PLUS jet nebulizer & Pulmo–Aide compressor	520	Lung function (FEV1) and density of *Pseudomonas aeruginosa in sputum*	At 6 months, nebulized tobramycin improved lung function, reduced hospitalizations and reduced sputum density of *Pseudomonas*
Konstan, 2010	Tobramycin powder 112 mg bid compared to tobramycin 300 mg bid	T-326 Inhaler: Dry powder inhaler PARI LC PLUS jet nebulizer & Pulmo–Aide compressor	553	Safety & efficacy: Lung function (FEV1), density of *Pseudomonas*, antibiotic use, administration time between nebulized tobramycin and DPI	At 24 weeks, DPI tobramycin had comparable safety and efficacy profile to nebulized tobramycin. DPI treatment time was less (5.6 min vs 19.7 min)
McCoy, 2008	Aztreonam lysine 75 mg bid – tid Administered on 28-day cycle	Pari LC PLUS jet nebulizer	246	Clinical worsening; time to need for additional anti-pseudomonal antibiotics for exacerbations	At 84 days of follow up, nebulized aztreonam delayed need for antibiotic therapy, improved lung function, symptoms and reduced sputum density of *Pseudomonas*
Schuster, 2012	Micronised Colistimethate 1,662,500 IU bid compared to tobramycin 300 mg bid	Dry powder inhaler Pari LC PLUS jet nebulizer with suitable compressor	380	Lung function (FEV1) from baseline at 24 weeks, adverse events, medication compliance	DPI colistimethate was non-inferior compared to nebulized tobramycin solution Cough and abnormal taste more frequent with colistimethate DPI

Abbreviations: FEV1 = forced expiratory volume in 1 second; DPI = dry powder inhaler.

Table 12.3: A Closer Look at Inhaled Delivery Systems

Device Name	Description	Instructions for Use
TOBI Podhaler	• Dry powder inhaler • Manufactured by BGP Products Operation GmbH (Vitaris), Steinhausen, Switzerland	• Store capsules in blister cards; remove only immediately before use • Wash and dry hands • Unscrew the lid and body of mouthpiece in counterclockwise direction • Place one capsule in chamber at top of podhaler device • Put mouthpiece back on and screw tightly in clockwise fashion • Press the blue button all the way down one time only • Breathe out all the way. Place mouth over mouthpiece with tight seal. Inhale deeply with single breath. Hold for 10 seconds, and exhale slowly • Repeat second inhalation using same capsule • Confirm used capsule is pierced and empty. Toss it away • Repeat three more times until full dose is taken • Wipe mouthpiece with clean cloth • Place lid back on and store at room temperature between 68 and 77 degrees Fahrenheit
Turbospin	• Dry powder inhaler • Manufactured by Forest Laboratories, New York, NY, USA	• Remove the cap and unscrew the mouthpiece • Insert capsule into chamber with widest end first • Put mouthpiece back on and screw tightly • To pierce the capsule, hold mouthpiece upright and gently push the piston upwards until the visible line is reached. This locks the capsule in place • Continue pushing the piston as far as it will go and then release. Do this only once • Breathe out all the way. Place mouth over mouthpiece with tight seal. Inhale deeply with single breath. Hold for 10 seconds, and exhale slowly • Repeat second inhalation using same capsule • Check capsule has been emptied. Rinse mouth with water • Unscrew mouthpiece, then remove and discard empty capsule
PARI eFlow	• Electronic nebulizer • Manufactured by PARI Innovative Manufacturers, Midlothian, VA, USA	• Pour medication into reservoir as prescribed. Do not overfill • Attach medication cap; it will snap audibly into place • Press cap down gently and twist it clockwise • Link nebulizer handset to control unit with connecting cord • Place mouth over mouthpiece. Press on/off button on the control unit to start generating the aerosol • The green LED lights up and emits a tone • Sit in an upright and relaxed position. Breathe in and out as deeply and calmly as possible through the mouthpiece • Keep the mouthpiece in your mouth even when exhaling. Avoid breathing through your nose • Always hold the handset horizontally • When completed, clean and disinfect the system after each use

twentieth century, clinical trials that examined the effect of inhaled antibiotics for the treatment of chronic *Pseudomonas* colonization in patients with CF showed promising results (Table 12.2) (30). An initial trial examined tobramycin delivery via ultrasonic nebulizer to stable patients with CF and reported improved lung function, reduced exacerbations, and decreased sputum density of *Pseudomonas* (31). A subsequent multicenter trial assessed the efficacy and safety of nebulized tobramycin over 6 months and demonstrated clinical benefits (Table 12.2) (32). Following these reports, FDA approval was granted for chronic maintenance therapy with inhaled tobramycin to patients with CF > 6 years of age. Inhaled tobramycin is formulated for use with a specific nebulizer/compressor PARI-LC PLUS jet nebulizer and DeVilbiss Pulmo-Aide compressor. The Pari-LC is a breath-enhanced nebulizer designed to provide more aerosolized medication during inhalation than on exhalation, an internal valve closes to route air out via the expiratory valve in the mouthpiece. This process results in greater aerosol containment in the nebulizer chamber leading to greater inhaled aerosol mass and reduction in loss to the ambient surroundings (33). A dry powder formulation of tobramycin is commercially available (TOBI Podhaler) that is well tolerated and reduces delivery time with similar clinical efficacy compared with the nebulized formulation (Table 12.3) (9).

Inhaled aztreonam was approved for CF patients with chronic *Pseudomonas* infection. Approval was based on clinical trials demonstrating improvements in lung function, symptoms and decreased density of Pseudomonas in sputum (Table 12.2) (34, 35). Aztreonam is delivered by vibrating mesh nebulization (75 mg) on a 28-day on, 28-day off cycle. Thrice daily dosing (75 mg) with a 28-day cycle is the optimal schedule (35, 36). Currently, inhaled aztreonam is approved for patients with CF ≥ 6 years of age and chronic *Pseudomonas* airway colonization. Inhaled colistimethate, a polymyxin version of colistin, is available as a solution for nebulization. In Europe, it is first-line therapy for the treatment of CF with chronic *Pseudomonas* infection. A dry powder formulation (Colobreathe) is available for use in Europe that delivers an emitted dose of 125 mg from a Turbospin device (Table 12.3; Figure 12.1).

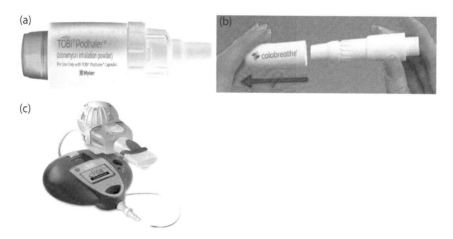

Figure 12.1 Devices employed for delivery of inhaled antibiotics: (a) TOBI Podhaler, dry powder inhaler; (b) Turbospin, dry powder inhaler; (c) Pari eFlow, electronic nebulizer.

Table 12.4: Inhaled Antibiotics for the Treatment of Non-cystic Fibrosis Bronchiectasis

Author and Publication Year	Drug Dose and Frequency	Delivery Device	Subjects (N)	Primary Outcome	Results
Barker, 2000	300 mg tobramycin bid	PARI LC PLUS jet nebulizer and a Pulmo-Aide compressor	74	*Pseudomonas aeruginosa* sputum density; lung function	Significant reduction in sputum *Pseudomonas aeruginosa* but no difference in lung function in nebulized tobramycin compared to placebo group
Barker, 2014	75 mg aztreonam lysin tid Administered on 28-day cycle	Pari LC PLUS jet nebulizer	AIRBX1: 266 AIRBX2: 274	Quality of Life- Bronchiectasis Respiratory Symptom scores and exacerbations	In two phase 3 trials (AIRBX1 & AIRBX2), nebulized aztreonam did not provide significant clinical benefit compared to placebo group
De Soyza, 2018	Ciprofloxacin dry powder inhaler 32.5 mg bid Administered on 14 or 28-day cycles	Dry powder inhaler	416	Time to first exacerbation and frequency of exacerbations	At 48 weeks, dry powder inhaler ciprofloxacin 14 days on/off cycle significantly delayed time to first exacerbation & reduced exacerbations compared to placebo; dry powder inhaler 28 days not different to placebo
Aksamit, 2018	Ciprofloxacin dry powder inhaler 32.5 mg bid Administered on 14 or 28-day cycles	Dry powder inhaler	521	Time to first exacerbation and frequency of exacerbations	At 48 weeks, 14- and 28-day dry powder inhaler ciprofloxacin cycles showed a trend for increased time to first exacerbation compared to placebo Neither treatment arm showed statistical significance in endpoints
Haworth, 2019	Liposomal ciprofloxacin 135 mg, ciprofloxacin 54 mg	PARI LC Sprint jet nebulizer	ORBIT3: 290 ORBIT4: 308	Time to first exacerbation	At 48 weeks, nebulized liposomal ciprofloxacin led to longer median time to first exacerbation compared to placebo in ORBIT-4 group but not in ORBIT-3 or pooled analysis
Haworth, 2014	Colistin 1 million IU	I-neb adaptive mesh nebulizer	144	Time to first exacerbation	Primary endpoint not reached Colistin increased time to first exacerbation but did not reach statistical significance compared to placebo

Abbreviations: IU = International units; tid = three times daily.

Table 12.5: Compatibility of Solutions/Suspensions Used Simultaneously with Jet Nebulizers

	Albuterol	Budesonide	Dornase Alfa	Ipratropium	Sodium Chloride (5.8%)	Tobramycin
Albuterol		NR	NR	C	NR	C
Budesonide	C		NR	C	C	C
Dornase alfa	NR	NR		NR	NR	NR
Ipratropium	C	C	NR		NR	C
Sodium chloride (5.8%)	NR	C	NR	NR		NR
Tobramycin	C	C	NR	NR	NR	

Abbreviations: C = compatible; NR = not recommended.

Note: (a) All solutions should be prepared from formulations without preservatives, (b) physical and chemical compatibilities do not predict the effects on aerosol aerodynamic behavior, (c) decreases in temperature can occur with nebulizers and investigations on compatibility are limited, (d) combining solutions can increase total chamber volume with diminished drug delivery. Modified from Burchett DK. Am J Health-Syst Pharm 2010 (45), Kamin W. J Cystic Fibrosis 2014 (46).

Clinical trials examining inhaled antibiotics in patients with NCFB have not demonstrated significant improvements in lung function, symptoms, or exacerbations (Table 12.4). Early clinical trials demonstrated reductions in airway bacterial density (37–39). Multicenter trials comparing clinical outcomes of dry powder and nebulized liposomal ciprofloxacin in patients with NCFB did not achieve their primary endpoints (Table 12.4) (40–42). A comprehensive meta-analysis reported a decrease in bacterial density and a small but statistically significant decrease in exacerbation rates without an improvement in quality of life (43). Concerns about the diversity of underlying causes of bronchiectasis, variation in exacerbation rate, and study design appear to influence the findings in the non-CF population. Currently, the European Respiratory Society and British Thoracic Society recommend inhaled antibiotics (colistin or gentamicin) for patients with ≥ 3 exacerbations/year with chronic *P. aeruginosa* airway infection (2, 44).

COMBINATIONS OF NEBULIZER SOLUTIONS

Inhalation therapy by jet nebulization can be time-consuming lasting 10 to 15 minutes per medication. To reduce drug delivery time, patients may combine drug solutions in a nebulizer chamber to shorten administration time. However, certain drug solutions should not be combined as this can lead to incompatibilities that may alter drug efficacy. Clinicians should be aware of these drug compatibilities and Table 12.5 provides guidance regarding the compatibility of various drug solutions for nebulization (45, 46).

CONCLUSION

Inhaled therapies are commonly employed in patients with bronchiectasis and have shown beneficial effects in patients with CF bronchiectasis. However, similar improvements in clinical outcomes with inhaled therapies have not been reported in patients with non-cystic fibrosis bronchiectasis.

REFERENCES

1. Imam JS, Duarte AG. Non-CF bronchiectasis: Orphan disease no longer. Respir Med 2020;166(105940):105940.
2. Polverino E, Goeminne PC, McDonnell MJ, et al. European Respiratory Society guidelines for the management of adult bronchiectasis. Eur Respir J 2017;50(3):1700629.
3. Cystic Fibrosis Foundation. Chronic medications to maintain lung health clinical care guidelines. [cited 2022 Jun 3]. Available from: https://www.cff.org/chronic-medications-maintain-lung-health-clinical-care-guidelines
4. Aksamit TR, O'Donnell AE, Barker A, et al. Adult patients with bronchiectasis: A first look at the US Bronchiectasis Research Registry. Chest 2017;151(5):982–992. DOI:10.1016/j.chest.2016.10.055
5. Franco F, Sheikh A, Greenstone M. Short acting beta-2 agonists for bronchiectasis. Cochrane Database Syst Rev 2003;(3):CD003572.
6. Martínez-García M, Oscullo G, García-Ortega A, et al. Rationale and clinical use of bronchodilators in adults with bronchiectasis. Drugs 2022;82(1):1–13.
7. Restrepo RD. Inhaled adrenergics and anticholinergics in obstructive lung disease: Do they enhance mucociliary clearance? Respir Care 2007;52(9):1159–1173; discussion 1173–1175.
8. Daniels T, Mills N, Whitaker P. Nebuliser systems for drug delivery in cystic fibrosis. Cochrane Database Syst Rev 2013;(4):CD007639.

9. Anderson PJ. Cystic fibrosis and bronchiectasis. In: Dhand R, editor. ISAM Textbook of Aerosol Medicine. Knoxville (TN): International Society for Aerosols in Medicine; 2016. p. e755–e780. ISBN 978-0-9963711-0-0.

10. Mogayzel PJ Jr, Naureckas ET, Robinson KA, et al. Cystic fibrosis pulmonary guidelines. Chronic medications for maintenance of lung health. Am J Respir Crit Care Med 2013;187(7):680–689. DOI:10.1164/rccm.201207-1160oe

11. Smyth AR, Bell SC, Bojcin S, et al. European cystic fibrosis society standards of care: Best practice guidelines. J Cyst Fibros 2014;13(Suppl 1):S23–S42.

12. Kapur N, Petsky HL, Bell S, et al. Inhaled corticosteroids for bronchiectasis. Cochrane Database Syst Rev 2018;5(5):CD000996.

13. Elborn JS, Johnston B, Allen F, et al. Inhaled steroids in patients with bronchiectasis. Respir Med 1992;86(2):121–124.

14. Hernando R, Drobnic ME, Cruz MJ, et al. Budesonide efficacy and safety in patients with bronchiectasis not due to cystic fibrosis. Int J Clin Pharm 2012;34(4):644–650.

15. Tsang KW, Ho PL, Lam WK, et al. Inhaled fluticasone reduces sputum inflammatory indices in severe bronchiectasis. Am J Respir Crit Care Med 1998;158(3):723–727.

16. Liu VX, Winthrop KL, Lu Y, et al. Association between inhaled corticosteroid use and pulmonary nontuberculous mycobacterial infection. Ann Am Thorac Soc 2018;15(10):1169–1176. DOI:10.1513/AnnalsATS.201804-245OC

17. Elkins MR, Robinson M, Rose BR, et al. A controlled trial of long-term inhaled hypertonic saline in patients with cystic fibrosis. N Engl J Med 2006;354(3):229–240. DOI:10.1056/NEJMoa043900

18. Wark P, McDonald VM. Nebulised hypertonic saline for cystic fibrosis. Cochrane Database Syst Rev 2009;(2):CD001506.

19. Kellett F, Robert NM. Nebulised 7% hypertonic saline improves lung function and quality of life in bronchiectasis. Respir Med 2011;105(12):1831–1835.

20. Nicolson CHH, Stirling RG, Borg BM, et al. The long term effect of inhaled hypertonic saline 6% in non-cystic fibrosis bronchiectasis. Respir Med 2012;106(5):661–667.

21. Nevitt SJ, Thornton J, Murray CS, et al. Inhaled mannitol for cystic fibrosis. Cochrane Database Syst Rev 2020;5(5):CD008649.

22. De Boeck K, Haarman E, Hull J, et al. Inhaled dry powder mannitol in children with cystic fibrosis: A randomised efficacy and safety trial. J Cyst Fibros 2017;16(3):380–387.

23. Bronchitol (mannitol) inhalation powder [Internet]. Fda.gov. [cited 2022 Jun 3]. Available from: https://www.accessdata.fda.gov/drugsatfda_docs/label/2020/202049s000lbl.pdf

24. Bilton D, Tino G, Barker AF, et al. Inhaled mannitol for non-cystic fibrosis bronchiectasis: A randomised, controlled trial. Thorax 2014;69(12):1073–1079.

25. Tarrant BJ, Le Maitre C, Romero L, et al. Mucoactive agents for chronic, non-cystic fibrosis lung disease: A systematic review and meta-analysis. Respirology 2017;22(6):1084–1092.

26. Tam J, Nash EF, Ratjen F, et al. Nebulized and oral thiol derivatives for pulmonary disease in cystic fibrosis. Cochrane Database Syst Rev 2013;2013(7):CD007168. DOI:10.1002/14651858.CD007168.pub3

27. Yang C, Montgomery M. Dornase alfa for cystic fibrosis. Cochrane Database Syst Rev 2021;3(3):CD001127. DOI:10.1002/14651858.CD001127.pub5

28. O'Donnell AE, Barker AF, Ilowite JS, et al. Treatment of idiopathic bronchiectasis with aerosolized recombinant human DNase i. rhDNase study group. Chest 1998;113(5):1329–1334.

29. Garthwaite B, Barach AL, Levenson E, et al. Penicillin aerosol therapy in bronchiectasis, lung abscess and chronic bronchitis [Internet]. Amjmed. com. 1947 [cited 2022 Jun 3]. Available from: https://www.amjmed.com/article/0002-9343(47)90158-7/fulltext

30. Quon BS, Goss CH, Ramsey BW. Inhaled antibiotics for lower airway infections. Ann Am Thorac Soc 2014;11(3):425–434.

31. Ramsey BW, Dorkin HL, Eisenberg JD, et al. Efficacy of aerosolized tobramycin in patients with cystic fibrosis. N Engl J Med 1993;328(24): 1740–1746. DOI:10.1056/NEJM199306173282403

32. Ramsey BW, Pepe MS, Quan JM, et al. Intermittent administration of inhaled tobramycin in patients with cystic fibrosis. Cystic Fibrosis Inhaled Tobramycin Study Group. N Engl J Med 1999;340(1):23–30. DOI:10.1056/NEJM199901073400104

33. Fink JB, Stapleton KW. Nebulizers. In: Dhand R, editor, ISAM textbook of aerosol medicine. Knoxville (TN): International Society for Aerosols in Medicine;2016. p. e617–e655. ISBN 978-0-9963711-0-0.

34. McCoy KS, Quittner AL, Oermann CM, et al. Inhaled aztreonam lysine for chronic airway *Pseudomonas aeruginosa* in cystic fibrosis. Am J Respir Crit Care Med 2008;178(9):921–928.

35. Retsch-Bogart GZ, Quittner AL, Gibson RL, et al. Efficacy and safety of inhaled aztreonam lysine for airway pseudomonas in cystic fibrosis. Chest 2009;135(5):1223–1232.

36. Oermann CM, Retsch-Bogart GZ, Quittner AL, et al. An 18-month study of the safety and efficacy of repeated courses of inhaled aztreonam lysine in cystic fibrosis. Pediatr Pulmonol 2010;45(11):1121–1134.

37. Barker AF, Couch L, Fiel SB, et al. Tobramycin solution for inhalation reduces sputum *Pseudomonas aeruginosa* density in bronchiectasis. Am J Respir Crit Care Med 2000;162(2 Pt 1):481–485.

38. Murray MP, Govan JRW, Doherty CJ, et al. A randomized controlled trial of nebulized gentamicin in non-cystic fibrosis bronchiectasis. Am J Respir Crit Care Med 2011;183(4):491–499.

39. Barker AF, O'Donnell AE, Flume P, et al. Aztreonam for inhalation solution in patients with non-cystic fibrosis bronchiectasis (AIR-BX1 and AIR-BX2): Two randomised double-blind, placebo-controlled phase 3 trials. Lancet Respir Med 2014;2(9):738–749.

40. De Soyza A, Aksamit T, Bandel T-J, et al. RESPIRE 1: A phase III placebo-controlled randomised trial of ciprofloxacin dry powder for inhalation in non-cystic fibrosis bronchiectasis. Eur Respir J 2018;51(1):1702052.

41. Aksamit T, De Soyza A, Bandel T-J, et al. RESPIRE 2: A phase III placebo-controlled randomised trial of ciprofloxacin dry powder for inhalation in non-cystic fibrosis bronchiectasis. Eur Respir J 2018;51(1):1702053.

42. Haworth CS, Bilton D, Chalmers JD, et al. Inhaled liposomal ciprofloxacin in patients with non-cystic fibrosis bronchiectasis and chronic lung infection with *Pseudomonas aeruginosa* (ORBIT-3 and ORBIT-4): Two phase 3, randomised controlled trials. Lancet Respir Med 2019;7(3):213–226.

43. Laska IF, Crichton ML, Shoemark A, et al. The efficacy and safety of inhaled antibiotics for the treatment of bronchiectasis in adults: A systematic review and meta-analysis. Lancet Respir Med 2019;7(10):855–869.
44. Hill AT, Sullivan AL, Chalmers JD, et al. British Thoracic Society Guideline for bronchiectasis in adults. Thorax 2019;74(Suppl 1):1–69.
45. Burchett DK, Darko W, Zahra J, et al. Mixing and compatibility guide for commonly used aerosolized medications [Internet]. Unboundmedicine. com. 2010 [cited 2022 Jun 3]. Available from: https://www. unboundmedicine.com/medline/citation/20101066/full_citation/Mixing_ and_compatibility_guide_for_commonly_used_aerosolized_medications_
46. Kamin W, Erdnüss F, Krämer I. Inhalation solutions–which ones may be mixed? Physico-chemical compatibility of drug solutions in nebulizers– update 2013. J Cyst Fibros 2014;13(3):243–250.

13 Inhaled Therapy for Other Respiratory Diseases

Pulmonary Hypertension

Isaac N. Biney and Francisco J. Soto

CONTENTS

INTRODUCTION

The 6th World Symposium on Pulmonary Hypertension (PH) organized by the World Health Organization defines PH as mean pulmonary artery pressure (mPAP) >20 mmHg measured during right heart catheterization (1). PH is classified into five groups: Group 1, pulmonary arterial hypertension (PAH); group 2, PH due to left heart disease; Group 3, PH related to lung disease and/or hypoxia; group 4, PH due to pulmonary artery obstructions; and group 5, PH with unclear or multifactorial mechanisms (1). In addition to mPAP >20 mmHg, group 1 PAH definition requires a pulmonary capillary wedge pressure ≤15 mmHg and pulmonary vascular resistance (PVR) ≥3 Wood units.

Available PH-specific therapies lead to vasodilation and inhibition of smooth muscle cell proliferation (2) and target one of three pathways central to endothelial function (Figure 13.1): prostacyclin, nitric oxide, and endothelin pathways (3). The Food and Drug Administration (FDA) has approved ten drugs for use in PH. Four of these are available for administration via the inhalational route (4) (Table 13.1). PH-specific therapies are currently indicated for group 1, group 4, and more recently, for a subset of group 3 secondary to interstitial lung disease (ILD) (5).

ADVANTAGES AND LIMITATIONS OF INHALED THERAPIES FOR PULMONARY HYPERTENSION

Delivering the drug directly to the site of disease allows for high local concentrations, reduces the risk of systemic side effects (6), and potentially decreases cost of treatment (7). Drug delivery to well-ventilated regions enhances blood flow and improves gas exchange (8). Inhaled route limitations include irritant effects on the airways (7), unpredictable breathing patterns affecting the exact dose of drug delivered (4), short half-life of the available therapies requiring frequent inhalations and longer inhalation time, and cumbersome use and maintenance of the delivery systems (9).

DOI: 10.1201/9781003269014-13

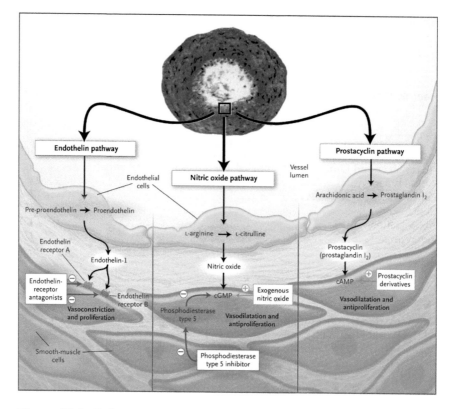

Figure 13.1 Pathway targets for current therapies in pulmonary arterial hypertension (PAH). The three major pathways involved in the pathophysiology of PAH; The prostacyclin pathway, nitric oxide pathway, and endothelin pathway are shown. The transverse section of a small pulmonary artery in a patient with PAH is shown at the top of the figure with intimal proliferation and medial hypertrophy. There is decreased production of prostacyclin and endogenous nitric oxide and increased production of endothelin-1. (From the New England Journal of Medicine, Marc Humbert, Olivier Sitbon, Gérald Simonneau, Treatment of Pulmonary Arterial Hypertension, volume 351, pages 1425–1436. Copyright © 2022 Massachusetts Medical Society. Reprinted with permission from Massachusetts Medical Society.)

PATHWAYS

Prostacyclin Pathway

Prostacyclin is a prostaglandin synthesized by vascular endothelial cells. It binds to receptors stimulating the production of cyclic adenosine monophosphate, promoting pulmonary artery vasodilation, and inhibiting vascular smooth muscle cell proliferation and platelet aggregation (10). Three prostacyclin analogs are available for inhaled delivery: iloprost (Ventavis®), treprostinil (Tyvaso®), and epoprostenol (Flolan®, Veletri®) (11).

Iloprost

Iloprost was the first prostacyclin analog approved for inhalation use (12). It is indicated for the treatment of group 1 PAH (13, 14). It requires 6–9 inhalations

Table 13.1: Formulation, Delivery Device, Dose, and Indications of Currently Available Inhaled Therapies for Pulmonary Hypertension

Drug	Brand Name (Manufacture)	Formulation	Delivery Device	Dose	Indication
Iloprost	Ventavis (Actelion Pharmaceuticals	Aerosol	I-neb AAD system	2.5 or 5 µg/dose 6–9 times/day	Group 1 PAH
Treprostinil	Tyvaso (United Therapeutics) Tyvaso DPI	Aerosol Dry powder	Opti-neb (Tyvaso inhalation system) Dry powder inhaler	3–12 puffs (18–72 µg)/dose 4 times/day 1 puff (16–64 µg)/dose 4 times/day	Group 1 PAH Group 3 PAH related to ILD
Epoprostenol	Flolan (GlaxoSmith Kline) Veletri (Actelion Pharmaceuticals)	Aerosol Aerosol	Vibrating mesh nebulizer Vibrating mesh nebulizer	10–50 ng/kg/min	Vasoreactivity testing[a] PH in critically ill patients[a]
Nitric oxide	N/A Vero biotech	Gas	Cylinder-based systems Genosyl DS Disposable cassette	5–40 ppm 1–80 ppm	Vasoreactivity testing[a] PH in critically ill patients[a]

[a] Off-label application.

Abbreviations: AAD = adaptive aerosol delivery, DPI = dry powder inhaler, DS = delivery system, ILD = interstitial lung disease, PAH = pulmonary arterial hypertension, PH = pulmonary hypertension.

a day of either 2.5 or 5 µg dose per treatment to maintain therapeutic levels (4) given its 20–30-minute half-life (15).

Efficacy

Iloprost approval for PAH was based on a study showing improvement in a combined endpoint of at least one New York Heart Association class and at least a 10% increase in 6-minute walk distance (6MWD) (16).

Delivery Devices

In the United States (US) and the European Union (EU), inhaled iloprost is administered using the I-neb adaptive aerosol delivery (AAD) system (Phillips Respironics Ltd., UK) (13, 17). This device is a small, portable, light, and quiet delivery system coupling a vibrating mesh nebulizer platform with AAD technology (Figure 13.2A). The I-neb AAD system delivers a precise dose by pulsing the aerosol during the first 50–80% of the inhalation and adapting the delivery to the patient's breathing pattern (18). Synchronization with inspiration helps avoid waste during exhalation and allows the dose delivered to be reasonably predicted (19). The performance of the I-neb AAD system has been confirmed by *in vitro* studies in which the measured delivered doses of the 2.5 and 5 µg metered iloprost doses were 2.8 and 4.9 µg, respectively (20). The I-neb device provides visual, auditory, and tactile

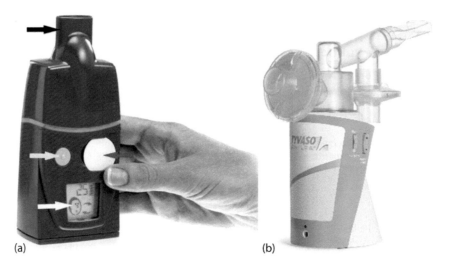

(a)   (b)

Figure 13.2   (a, b) The I-neb adaptive aerosol delivery system (a) showing the
on button (yellow arrow), display screen (white arrow), dosing disc (red arrow),
and the mouthpiece (black arrow). (Republished with permission of Daedalus
Enterprises Inc., from inhaled therapies for pulmonary hypertension, Hill
et al., Respiratory Care, volume 60, issue 6, ©2015), and the TYVASO inhalation
system. (b) The run/program switch allows the patient to set the number of
breaths and deliver the dose. The volume/breaths toggle button increases or
decreases the volume of the prompts or the number of breaths to be delivered
when the switch is set to run or program, respectively. (Used with permission.
©2022 United Therapeutics Corporation.)

feedback after each inhalation and after the programmed dose is completed.
Moreover, it can also monitor patient adherence (19). Disadvantages of the
I-neb device include the time for each treatment (up to 10 minutes) and the
need for thorough cleaning after each use to maintain the function of the
vibrating mesh (21, 22). Instructions for using the I-neb are shown in
Table 13.2.

BREELIB™ (Vectura Group plc Chippenham, UK) is a recently introduced
nebulizer. Iloprost delivery with BREELIB™ was well tolerated in a recent study
of PAH patients with the delivery of 5 µg of iloprost in a median duration of
2.6 minutes (21). The BREELIB™ has a vibrating mesh aerosol generator that
offers a breath-triggered aerosol bolus followed by aerosol-free air. The speed
of inhalation is restricted by a mechanical flow-limitation valve and feedback
is provided when the target inhalation volume is reached. This ensures the
delivery of an exact and reproducible dose (22). It was approved in the EU
in 2016. Recent data confirmed its ability to provide an acute hemodynamic
response with delivery of iloprost (23).

Treprostinil

Treprostinil can be administered via subcutaneous, intravenous (IV), inhaled,
and oral routes (24). Inhaled treprostinil (iTRE) is indicated for the treatment of
group 1 PAH and group 3 ILD-related PH (14, 25). It is administered four times
daily and is the most stable of the prostacyclin analogues, with hemodynamic
effects observed beyond 3 hours post-inhalation (26).

Table 13.2: Instructions for Using the I-neb Adaptive Aerosol Delivery (AAD) System and the Tyvaso Inhalation System

Device	Instructions
I-neb AAD system	1. Charge the battery for 3–6 hours 2. Insert the prescribed dosing disc 3. Assemble the device 4. Turn on the device and wait until the start-up screen appears which will show the dose about to be taken 5. Hold the I-neb horizontally with the display screen facing down 6. Seal your lips around the mouthpiece and breathe in and out through your mouth 7. After a few breaths, the device will start delivering a medication, this will be felt as a vibration with each breath 8. Continue to breathe through the device until the buzzer is heard which indicates treatment is complete 9. Removing the mouthpiece from the mouth will pause the treatment
Tyvaso inhalation system	1. The prescribed number of breaths should be set 2. Load the medication cup and assemble the device 3. Power on the device, if the internal battery is too low to deliver the full treatment, plug in the device 4. Hold the device upright, the display screen should be visible, and avoid covering the bottom of the device so the audio speaker is not blocked 5. Push the start button, when prompted, exhale to prepare to inhale 6. When prompted to inhale, place lips securely around the mouthpiece and inhale for 3 seconds. When the lights stop flashing, remove the lips from the mouthpiece and exhale normally 7. Repeat for each remaining breath

Abbreviation: AAD = adaptive aerosol delivery

Efficacy

iTRE approval for group 1 PAH was based on a trial showing improvement in 6MWD, pro-brain natriuretic peptide and quality of life (27). Approval for use in group 3, ILD-related PH was based on a recent study showing improvement in 6MWD (28).

Delivery Devices

iTRE is administered with the Tyvaso inhalation system (Figure 13.2B), the Opti-Neb-ir Model ON-100/7 (Nebu-Tec, Elsenfeld, Germany) (29). This is a hand-held ultrasonic, pulsed delivery device delivering approximately 6 µg of treprostinil per breath (24). The medication is initiated at a dose of 3 breaths (18 µg) four times daily. The maintenance goal is 9–12 breaths (54–72 µg) per dose (30), delivered in 2–3 minutes (31). The system's display screen indicates the programmed number of breaths and breaths left in the current dose, prompts the patient to inhale and exhale, and informs when the treatment session is complete. It requires daily assembly and cleaning, and its maintenance can be burdensome (31). Instructions for using the Tyvaso inhalation system are shown in Table 13.2.

iTRE is also available in a dry powder inhalation (DPI) formulation (32, 33). The FDA recently approved the Tyvaso DPI (United Therapeutics/MannKind Corporation, US) which was shown to be safe and well tolerated (34). The cartridges come in four different strengths (16, 32, 48, and 64 µg) which allows dose titration. The cartridge is inserted into the device and the dose is delivered in one inhalation (35). Another DPI formulation is the LIQ861 (Liquidia, North Carolina, US), an investigational DPI using PRINT® technology to enhance deep-lung delivery and enable drug administration in 1–2 breaths (31, 36, 37) that is currently awaiting FDA approval.

Epoprostenol

Epoprostenol was the first FDA-approved prostacyclin for PAH, based on a trial demonstrating improved exercise tolerance, hemodynamics, and survival compared to conventional therapy (7, 38). Epoprostenol is the least stable of the prostacyclins. Its half-life is 3–5 minutes and is administered by continuous IV infusion (39, 40). The IV formulation can be aerosolized and used therapeutically off-label. However, it requires continuous nebulization due to its short half-life, making it impractical for long-term use (4, 7).

Drug Delivery and Efficacy

Vibrating mesh nebulizers are used to administer inhaled epoprostenol (iEPO), with no delivery system specifically designed for this purpose (41, 42). Jet nebulizers have been used but their inherent properties affect dose delivery (43). In mechanically ventilated patients, the vibrating mesh nebulizer is placed within the inspiratory limb, or at the humidifier inlet or outlet. Placement at the humidifier inlet/outlet results in higher drug deposition. Placement at the inlet prevents variability of drug deposition with tidal volume (Figure 13.3) (41). iEPO can also be delivered to patients on non-invasive positive pressure ventilation (NIPPV) and on high-flow nasal cannula (HFNC). The nebulizer is connected to the distal end of the NIPPV circuit and on the dry side of the

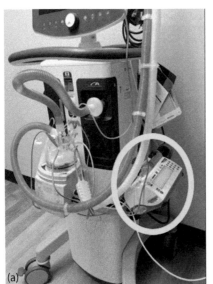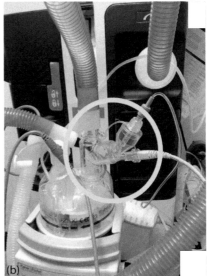

Figure 13.3   (a, b) Medfusion 3500 syringe pump (aqua circle 3a) used to deliver epoprostenol solution using a vibrating mesh nebulizer (aqua circle 3b) placed at the humidifier inlet (dry side) in a mechanical ventilation circuit.

HFNC humidifier (44, 45). If delivered with HFNC, the inhaled dose is higher when gas flow is set below the patient's inspiratory flow (46).

iEPO has been shown to consistently reduce pulmonary arterial pressures (PAP) in patients undergoing cardiac surgery, heart and lung transplantation, and patients with nonspecific critical illnesses. The clinical significance of these findings is unknown (47). In critically ill patients, continuous administration of epoprostenol allows for dose titration (48).

Nitric Oxide Pathway

Nitric oxide (NO) is a highly diffusible gas produced by vascular endothelial cells. It binds to and activates soluble guanylate cyclase resulting in vasodilation. It also inhibits platelet aggregation and has antiproliferative and anti-inflammatory effects (4). Given its very short half-life (seconds), it can be delivered by inhalation to exert local effects on the pulmonary vasculature with little or no systemic absorption (49).

Inhaled Nitric Oxide

Inhaled NO (iNO) is only approved for the treatment of PAH in newborns in both the US and EU. In adults, iNO is used off-label for vasoreactivity testing during the hemodynamic assessment of PAH patients (1).

Drug Delivery and Efficacy

iNO is used in cardiac surgery and in heart or lung transplantation, decreasing PAP and PVR with effects similar to iEPO (50). Small uncontrolled studies have examined the long-term use of iNO in pediatric and adult patients, but no large, randomized trials are available (51–55). Drawbacks to the use of iNO include its cost and rebound PH crises from abrupt discontinuation (7).

Most available iNO delivery systems are cylinder-based with pressurized NO buffered with an inert gas. They can deliver iNO continuously or in a pulsed fashion synced with respiration (56). iNO can be administered to mechanically ventilated patients and to spontaneously breathing patients by either face mask or nasal prongs (7, 56). The concentration of nitrogen dioxide (NO_2), a toxic metabolite, is monitored to ensure safe levels are maintained. The FDA has recently approved the Genosyl delivery system (Vero Biotech, Atlanta, Georgia: https://www.vero-biotech.com/) a portable device that generates NO from NO_2 using an ascorbic acid cartridge (56).

CONCLUSION

Drug administration by the inhalational route for PAH offers unique advantages by delivering medication directly to the pulmonary vasculature. Iloprost and treprostinil are approved for the management of PAH currently delivered by nebulization. Time required for treatment administration and maintenance of the delivery device are major drawbacks of the currently available systems. The recent introduction of a DPI formulation of treprostinil may help mitigate some of the challenges. Epoprostenol and nitric oxide are used off-label in the inpatient setting but the need for continuous administration is a major limitation for chronic management of PAH.

ABBREVIATIONS

FDA   Food and Drug Administration
HFNC   High-flow nasal cannula
iEPO   Inhaled epoprostenol
ILD   Interstitial lung disease

iNO   Inhaled nitric oxide
iTRE   Inhaled treprostinil
IV   Intravenous
mPAP   Mean pulmonary artery pressure
NIPPV   Non-invasive positive pressure ventilation
NO   Nitric oxide
PAH   Pulmonary arterial hypertension
PH   Pulmonary hypertension
PVR   Pulmonary vascular resistance
US   United States
WU   Wood units

REFERENCES

1. Simonneau G, Montani D, Celermajer DS. et al. Haemodynamic definitions and updated clinical classification of pulmonary hypertension. Eur Respir J 2019;53(1):1801913.
2. Sommer N, Ghofrani HA, Pak O. et al. Current and future treatments of pulmonary arterial hypertension. Br J Pharmacol 2021;178(1):6–30.
3. Galiè N, Channuck RN, Frantz RP. et al. Risk stratification and medical therapy of pulmonary arterial hypertension. Eur Respir J 2019;53(1):1801889.
4. Keshavarz A, Kadry H, Alobaida A. et al. Newer approaches and novel drugs for inhalational therapy for pulmonary arterial hypertension. Expert Opin Drug Deliv 2020;17(4):439–461.
5. Saunders H, Helgeson SA, Abdelrahim A. et al. Comparing diagnosis and treatment of pulmonary hypertension patients at a pulmonary hypertension center versus community centers. Diseases 2022;10(1):5.
6. Labiris NR, Dolovich MB. Pulmonary drug delivery. Part I: Physiological factors affecting therapeutic effectiveness of aerosolized medications. Br J Clin Pharmacol 2003;56(6):588–599.
7. Hill NS, Preston IR, Roberts KE. Inhaled therapies for pulmonary hypertension. Respir Care 2015;60(6):794–802; discussion 802–805.
8. Baradia D, Khatri N, Trehan S. et al. Inhalation therapy to treat pulmonary arterial hypertension. Pharm Pat Anal 2012;1(5):577–588.
9. Gessler T. Inhalation of repurposed drugs to treat pulmonary hypertension. Adv Drug Deliv Rev 2018;133:34–44.
10. Mandras S, Kovacs G, Olschewski H. et al. Combination therapy in pulmonary arterial hypertension-targeting the nitric oxide and prostacyclin pathways. J Cardiovasc Pharmacol Ther 2021;26(5):453–462.
11. Liu K, Wang H, Yu SJ. et al. Inhaled pulmonary vasodilators: A narrative review. Ann Transl Med 2021;9(7):597.
12. McLaughlin VV, Palevsky HI. Parenteral and inhaled prostanoid therapy in the treatment of pulmonary arterial hypertension. Clin Chest Med 2013;34(4):825–840.
13. Ventavis [package insert]. San Francisco (CA): Actelion Pharmaceuticals US, Inc.; 2019.
14. Galiè N, Humbert M, Vachiery JL. et al. 2015 ESC/ERS guidelines for the diagnosis and treatment of pulmonary hypertension: The joint task force for the diagnosis and treatment of pulmonary hypertension of the European Society of Cardiology (ESC) and the European Respiratory

Society (ERS): Endorsed by: Association for European Paediatric and Congenital Cardiology (AEPC), International Society for Heart and Lung Transplantation (ISHLT). Eur Respir J 2015;46(4): 903–975.

15. Hoeper MM, Schwarze M, Ehlerding S. et al. Long-term treatment of primary pulmonary hypertension with aerosolized iloprost, a prostacyclin analogue. N Engl J Med 2000;342(25):1866–1870.

16. Olschewski H, Simonneau G, Galie N. et al. Inhaled iloprost for severe pulmonary hypertension. N Engl J Med 2002;347(5):322–329.

17. Ventavis [package insert]. Madrid (Spain): Poligono Industrial Santa Rosa; 2021.

18. Hardaker LE, Hatley RH. In vitro characterization of the I-neb Adaptive Aerosol Delivery (AAD) system. J Aerosol Med Pulm Drug Deliv 2010;23(Suppl 1):S11–S20.

19. Dhand R. Intelligent nebulizers in the age of the Internet: The I-neb Adaptive Aerosol Delivery (AAD) system. J Aerosol Med Pulm Drug Deliv 2010;23(Suppl 1):iii–v.

20. Van Dyke RE, Nikander K. Delivery of iloprost inhalation solution with the HaloLite, Prodose, and I-neb Adaptive Aerosol Delivery systems: An in vitro study. Respir Care 2007;52(2):184–190.

21. Gessler T, Ghofrani HA, Held M. et al. The safety and pharmacokinetics of rapid iloprost aerosol delivery via the BREELIB nebulizer in pulmonary arterial hypertension. Pulm Circ 2017;7(2): 505–513.

22. Gessler T. Iloprost delivered via the BREELIB(TM) nebulizer: A review of the clinical evidence for efficacy and safety. Ther Adv Respir Dis 2019;13:1753466619835497.

23. Richter MJ, Wan J, Ghofrani HA. et al. Acute response to rapid iloprost inhalation using the Breelib™ nebulizer in pulmonary arterial hypertension: The Breelib™ acute study. Pulm Circ 2019;9(3):2045894019875342.

24. Kumar P, Thudium E, Laliberte K. et al. A comprehensive review of treprostinil pharmacokinetics via four routes of administration. Clin Pharmacokinet 2016;55(12):1495–1505.

25. Tyvaso [package insert]. Research Triangle Park (NC): United Therapeutics Corp.; 2021.

26. Voswinckel R, Enke B, Reichenberger F. et al. Favorable effects of inhaled treprostinil in severe pulmonary hypertension: Results from randomized controlled pilot studies. J Am Coll Cardiol 2006;48(8):1672–1681.

27. McLaughlin VV, Benza RL, Rubin LJ. et al. Addition of inhaled treprostinil to oral therapy for pulmonary arterial hypertension: A randomized controlled clinical trial. J Am Coll Cardiol 2010;55(18):1915–1922.

28. Waxman A, Restrepo-Jaramillo R, Thenappan T. et al. Inhaled treprostinil in pulmonary hypertension due to interstitial lung disease. N Engl J Med 2021;384(4):325–334.

29. Channick RN, Voswinckel R, Rubin LJ. Inhaled treprostinil: A therapeutic review. Drug Des Devel Ther 2012;6:19–28.

30. Soto FJ, Kravitz JN, Dhand R. Inhaled treprostinil in group 3 pulmonary hypertension. N Engl J Med 2021;384(19):1869–1870.

31. Roscigno RF, Vaughn T, Parsley E. et al. Comparative bioavailability of inhaled treprostinil administered as LIQ861 and Tyvaso® in healthy subjects. Vascul Pharmacol 2021;138: 106840.

32. Voswinckel R, Reichenberger F, Gall H. et al. Metered dose inhaler delivery of treprostinil for the treatment of pulmonary hypertension. Pulm Pharmacol Ther 2009;22(1):50–56.
33. Feldman J, Habib N, Fann J. et al. Treprostinil in the treatment of pulmonary arterial hypertension. Future Cardiol 2020;16(6):547–558.
34. Spikes L, Bajwa AA, Burger CD. et al. BREEZE: Open-label, clinical study to evaluate the safety and tolerability of a treprostinil dry powder inhaler in patients with pulmonary arterial hypertension currently using Tyvaso. Eur Respir J 2021;58(Suppl 65):PA1928.
35. Tyvaso DPI [package insert]. Research Triangle Park (NC): United Therapeutics/MannKind Corporation; 2022.
36. Hill NS, Feldman JP, Sahay S. et al. INSPIRE: A phase 3 open-label, multicenter study to evaluate the safety and tolerability of LIQ861 in pulmonary arterial hypertension (PAH) (Investigation of the safety and pharmacology of dry powder inhalation of treprostinil NCT03399604). J Heart Lung Transp 2019;38(11):S11.
37. Roscigno R, Vaughn T, Anderson S. et al. Pharmacokinetics and tolerability of LIQ861, a novel dry-powder formulation of treprostinil. Pulm Circ 2020;10(4):2045894020971509.
38. Barst RJ, Rubin LJ, Long WA. et al. A comparison of continuous intravenous epoprostenol (prostacyclin) with conventional therapy for primary pulmonary hypertension. N Engl J Med 1996;334(5):296–301.
39. Velitri [package insert]. San Francisco (CA): Actelion Pharmaceuticals US Inc.; 2021.
40. Flolan [package insert]. Research Triangle Park (NC): GlaxoSmithKline; 2021.
41. Anderson AC, Dubosky MN, Fiorino KA. et al. The effect of nebulizer position on aerosolized epoprostenol delivery in an adult lung model. Respir Care 2017;62(11):1387–1395.
42. Li J, Augustynovich AE, Gurnani PK, et al. In-vitro and in-vivo comparisons of high versus low concentrations of inhaled epoprostenol to adult intubated patients. Respir Res 2021;22(1):231.
43. Siobal M. Aerosolized prostacyclins. Respir Care 2004;49(6):640–652.
44. Ammar MA, Sasidhar M, Lam SW. Inhaled epoprostenol through noninvasive routes of ventilator support systems. Ann Pharmacother 2018;52(12):1173–1181.
45. Li J, Harnois LJ, Markos B. et al. Epoprostenol delivered via high flow nasal cannula for ICU subjects with severe hypoxemia comorbid with pulmonary hypertension or right heart dysfunction. Pharmaceutics 2019;11(6):281.
46. Li J, Gurnani PK, Roberts KM. et al. The clinical impact of flow titration on epoprostenol delivery via high flow nasal cannula for ICU patients with pulmonary hypertension or right ventricular dysfunction: A retrospective cohort comparison study. J Clin Med 2020;9(2):464.
47. Buckley MS, Feldman JP. Inhaled epoprostenol for the treatment of pulmonary arterial hypertension in critically ill adults. Pharmacotherapy 2010;30(7):728–740.
48. Muzevich KM, Chohan H, Grinnan DC. Management of pulmonary vasodilator therapy in patients with pulmonary arterial hypertension during critical illness. Crit Care 2014;18(5):523.
49. Abman SH. Inhaled nitric oxide for the treatment of pulmonary arterial hypertension. Handb Exp Pharmacol 2013;218:257–276.

50. Rao V, Ghadimi K, Keeyapaj W. et al. Inhaled nitric oxide (iNO) and inhaled epoprostenol (iPGI(2)) use in cardiothoracic surgical patients: Is there sufficient evidence for evidence-based recommendations? J Cardiothorac Vasc Anesth 2018;32(3):1452–1457.

51. Ivy DD, Parker D, Doran A. et al. Acute hemodynamic effects and home therapy using a novel pulsed nasal nitric oxide delivery system in children and young adults with pulmonary hypertension. Am J Cardiol 2003;92(7):886–890.

52. Pérez-Peñate GM, Juliá-Serdà G, Ojeda-Betancort N. et al. Long-term inhaled nitric oxide plus phosphodiesterase 5 inhibitors for severe pulmonary hypertension. J Heart Lung Transplant 2008;27(12):1326–1332.

53. Barst RJ, Channick R, Ivy D. et al. Clinical perspectives with long-term pulsed inhaled nitric oxide for the treatment of pulmonary arterial hypertension. Pulm Circ 2012;2(2):139–147.

54. Channick RN, Newhart JW, Johnson FW. et al. Pulsed delivery of inhaled nitric oxide to patients with primary pulmonary hypertension: An ambulatory delivery system and initial clinical tests. Chest 1996;109(6):1545–1549.

55. Preston IR, Klinger JR, Landzberg MJ, et al. Vasoresponsiveness of sarcoidosis-associated pulmonary hypertension. Chest 2001;120(3):866–872.

56. Gianni S, Carroll RW, Kacmarek RM. et al. Inhaled nitric oxide delivery systems for mechanically ventilated and nonintubated patients: A review. Respir Care 2021;66(6):1021–1028.

14 Regulatory Considerations Related to Inhaled Delivery Systems

Lydia I. Gilbert-McClain

CONTENTS

INTRODUCTION

The development of inhalation drugs for asthma and COPD has many advantages from both a safety and efficacy perspective. The inhaled route of administration allows for target delivery of the therapeutic to the site of action with the advantage of conferring efficacy while limiting systemic exposure and adverse effects. The advent of inhaled corticosteroids for the management of asthma is a clear example of the advantages of the inhaled route of delivery versus the systemic route of administration. Corticosteroids were first used to treat asthma in the 1950s (1). As a chronic inflammatory condition, the benefits of corticosteroids for the management of asthma are without question; however, the adverse effects of prolonged use of systemic corticosteroids were a limiting factor for its regular use in the maintenance treatment of asthma. The advent of corticosteroid drug products delivered via the inhaled route has the benefit of delivering effective therapies at significantly lower doses with resultant reduced systemic exposure and side effects. These advantages allowed for the use of corticosteroids for the maintenance treatment across the spectrum of asthma severity (mild to severe disease).

Efficacy of inhaled corticosteroids (ICS) for asthma was first reported in an article published in the Lancet in 1972 in which the author described inhaled beclomethasone having efficacy for the treatment of asthma with lesser adverse effects than systemic corticosteroids (2). In 1976, the first inhaled corticosteroid Vanceril (beclomethasone dipropionate, SCHERING) [now discontinued] was approved by the United States Food and Drug Administration (FDA) (3). Numerous single-ingredient ICS products have since been approved as well as fixed-dosed combination products of inhaled corticosteroids in combination with long-acting inhaled bronchodilators.

Since the first introduction of metered-dose inhalers in the late 1950s, many orally inhaled products including single-ingredient and fixed-dose combination products have been approved for asthma and COPD in a number of different devices and various formulations. As with all new

DOI: 10.1201/9781003269014-14

drugs, the demonstration of adequate evidence of efficacy and safety is necessary to support the approval of a new drug product by the FDA and the statutory requirements for drug development and approval are set forth in the Code of Federal Regulations (4). Because inhalation products incorporate a device, they are drug-device combination products, and both components, the device and the drug formulation constitute the drug product. Evidence of efficacy and safety must support not only the drug formulation but the efficacy and safety of the entire product. This means that the drug development program for each inhalation product is expected to generate data that provide information regarding all aspects of the product's clinical performance.

In this chapter, the regulatory considerations that impact the efficacy and safety of inhalation products are discussed. Regulatory issues for the development of generic products are not discussed in this chapter. Development of the generics of these complex dosage forms has unique considerations that are not the focus of this chapter. The FDA publishes product-specific guidance to provide recommendations to drug companies developing generics of orally inhaled products. The reader is referred to the FDA website on Product-Specific Guidance for further information on generic drug development (5).

DEVICE CONSIDERATIONS: DATA REQUIREMENTS

Consistent with its mission of promoting public health by providing safe and effective medicines for the American people, consumers can be assured that all inhaled products approved for marketing have undergone rigorous testing such that the product has met the statutory requirements to assure the safety and efficacy of the product for its intended use as described in the labeling for the product. Because device changes can have a significant impact on the safety and efficacy of drug-device combination products, as a general rule, drug developers use the product intended for marketing in their clinical studies and this would include not just their pivotal studies but the early dose-ranging studies. Several factors, including the drug substance, (i.e., the active pharmaceutical ingredient), the excipients (if any), and formulation and device characteristics may impact overall product performance and as a result the efficacy and safety of the product.

Device performance and formulation attributes for pressurized metered-dose inhalers (pMDIs) and dry powder inhalers (DPIs) are described in an FDA guidance document that provides information on the data necessary to support the performance of the drug product including the formulation and the device components. Among the many Chemistry, Manufacturing, and Controls (CMC) considerations needed to ensure the safety and efficacy of the product is the assurance that the drug product performance is such that the product delivers the correct therapeutic doses of drug substances consistently throughout the proposed shelf life of the product (6).

Several considerations influence the amount of data drug developers need to provide to demonstrate the adequate performance of their drug product. Factors such as the extent of previous regulatory experience with the active pharmaceutical ingredient(s) (API (s)), novel excipients in the formulation, and the device being used in the drug product can significantly impact the quantity of data needed to be generated to support a new drug product. For example, when a manufacturer develops a new drug product that incorporates a previously approved device, and that contains an active pharmaceutical ingredient already approved in an inhalation product the amount of data needed to be generated would generally be less. An example of this concept can be seen with the DPI single-ingredient, fixed-dose dual-ingredient, and fixed-dose triple-ingredient ELLIPTA products developed by GlaxoSmithKline. The ELLIPTA device is designed with two foil blister strips. Each blister strip contains the dry powder formulation [the single-ingredient products containing the active ingredient on each strip, the dual-ingredient products containing one active ingredient on each strip, and the triple ingredient product containing two of the active ingredients on one strip and the other active ingredient on one strip]. Delivery of the dose from the device involves the opening/turning of the inhalation mouthpiece which makes the dose ready for oral inhalation allowing the patient to receive the aerosolized formulation (7).

The first of these products approved was BREO ELLIPTA (fluticasone furoate and vilanterol inhalation powder, GlaxoSmithKline, Research Triangle Park, NC) a fixed-dose combination of an ICS (fluticasone furoate) and a long-acting beta-agonist (vilanterol). With the subsequent approval of the other ELLIPTA products, the FDA CMC reviews acknowledged the prior products' approval in the same device, and where appropriate the presence of a previously approved active ingredient. For example, with the FDA CMC regulatory considerations for the approval of ANORO ELLIPTA (umeclidinium bromide and vilanterol inhalation powder), the FDA CMC reviewer acknowledges the prior approval of vilanterol as part of the BREO ELLIPTA new drug application (8).

Another consideration that impacts the quantity of data needed with respect to device issues is that clinical tolerability data from any specific formulation or device may not be directly inferred from another. SPIRIVA® HANDIHALER® (tiotropium bromide inhalation powder, Boehringer Ingelheim Pharmaceuticals, Inc. Ridgefield, CT) was approved in 2004 for COPD. A new formulation of tiotropium bromide SPIRIVA® RESPIMAT® was subsequently developed for COPD and approved in 2014. Although the same active ingredient was present in both of these products, this change in formulation and device necessitated that the drug developer provide new data to support the tolerability of the new formulation, and the performance of the new device, as part of the overall evaluation of the safety and efficacy of the new product for the intended population.

The development of a new drug product that incorporates a new device not previously approved would need more extensive clinical data to support the safety of the product and in particular the robustness of the device. For conditions like asthma and COPD, where typically these therapies are used chronically, assurance of device functionality over repetitive use is essential. Further, approval of a product with a new device that had never been marketed previously raises questions about how the device would function in patients' hands overall. While clinical trials have limitations in addressing all the potential concerns that could ensue with a brand-new device, regulators are intentional about evaluating device robustness and patient-related issues that may pose a problem when new products are placed on the market. The goal of dedicated patient acceptance studies, and human factors engineering throughout the development program, is to ensure a high likelihood of success so that the interface between approved drug products and consumers would be as smooth as possible. Most of these evaluations to assess device robustness and functionality in patients' hands take place as part of the pivotal clinical trials and long-term safety trials where the effects of the formulation with chronic use can be evaluated, and device performance over the life of the device can be observed over a number of life cycles in a larger number of patients.

For example, the approval of the first RESPIMAT product COMBIVENT® RESPIMAT® (Ipratropium bromide and albuterol, Boehringer Ingelheim Pharmaceuticals, Inc., Ridgefield, CT) inhalation spray, the FDA required long-term safety data to evaluate the performance of the device over time. The approval of Combivent® Respimat® was introducing a brand-new inhalation device into the marketplace for which there was no prior real-world experience. The RESPIMAT® product comprises of two parts: a cartridge containing the formulation in solution and the inhalation device (the Respimat inhaler). The cartridge must first be inserted into the inhaler in order to use the product. Once inserted into the inhaler the cartridge is not removed. The device uses mechanical energy to generate a slow-moving aerosol cloud of medication from a metered volume of the drug solution. Prior to first use, the inhaler must be primed by actuating the inhaler toward the ground until an aerosol cloud is visible and then repeating the process three more times (9).

In the initial new drug application (NDA) submission, the product manufacturer provided data from two pivotal studies of 12-week treatment duration to support the efficacy and safety of the product. The active ingredients of the product ipratropium bromide and albuterol are well-known bronchodilators previously approved in other inhalation dosage forms as single-ingredient and combination products and the safety profile of these moieties is well established. As such, absent a new device, 12-week studies ordinarily may have been sufficient to support efficacy and safety. However, from the FDA's assessment, data from 12-week duration studies were insufficient to assess the long-term performance of a brand-new device. The application was not approved in the initial cycle due to inadequate long-term safety data and the lack of patients' use and handling information for the new drug delivery platform (10). In contrast to Combivent inhalation aerosol, [a standard press and breathe pMDI] that had been on the market for a long time and was a familiar device for patients, the new Respimat product was introducing a device for which there was no prior real-world experience. The Combivent Respimat product was intended to be a replacement product for the then-marketed Combivent inhalation aerosol (a pMDI product propelled by chlorofluorocarbons) and intended for long-term use. The FDA requested data to evaluate the long-term device robustness and performance and patient usability and acceptability as a requirement to support approval (11, 12). The company conducted a 48-week long-term safety and patient acceptability study that focused on the evaluation of device performance and patient acceptability of the Respimat product compared to the Combivent pMDI and albuterol and ipratropium bromide pMDI products (12).

An example of product changes that led to patient complaints was seen with the introduction of the more environment-friendly albuterol pMDIs propelled by hydrofluoroalkanes (HFA) to replace pMDIs propelled by the ozone-depleting chlorofluorocarbons (CFCs). Initially, many patients complained that the medication was not getting into their lungs and voiced concerns regarding the efficacy of these products as well as complaints regarding the taste and "feel" of the products (13). Differences between pMDIs propelled by CFC and pMDIs propelled by HFA contributed to these initial complaints as the spray from HFA-propelled pMDIs felt softer than the spray from CFC pMDIs. Subsequently,

FDA posted a "Frequently Asked Questions" page on its website to address complaints about the transition from CFC-propelled albuterol inhalers to HFA-propelled albuterol inhalers. The data from clinical trials with these products confirmed the efficacy of the HFA albuterol inhalers (14). Regular cleaning of the actuator and mouthpiece of HFA inhalers to prevent clogging of the inhaler orifice as well as being mindful of the priming instructions for these inhalers were differences that consumers had to adapt to with the transition to HFA-propelled pMDI inhalers. The labels for these HFA products note the importance of proper washing in that the inhaler may cease to deliver the medication if not thoroughly cleaned and dried (15).

FORMULATION CONSIDERATIONS

Patients with asthma and COPD characteristically have underlying airway hyperreactivity and may be particularly sensitive to minor changes in a formulation or device. Consequently, paradoxical bronchospasm is a potential safety concern with inhaled products in this population. The Full Prescribing Information for all orally inhaled products for asthma and COPD include a general warning statement about the potential for paradoxical bronchospasm. Impurities in the formulation must be tightly controlled. For pMDIs, potential sources of impurities can be from compounds that leach from elastomeric or plastic components, or coatings of the container and closure system as a result of direct contact with the formulation. FDA through years of experience with these products has acquired a wealth of knowledge regarding such potential impurities (16) and FDA guidance documents provide recommendations for the evaluation of leachables [and extractables] and for setting limits for levels of such impurities in drug product formulations (6).

Although DPIs are more complex device/container closure systems than pMDIs, the potential for leachables is significantly reduced because the drug product formulation in the DPI is [by definition] a dry powder and, unlike pMDIs, does not contain solvent systems such as organic propellants and co-solvents which can facilitate leaching. Dry powder formulations, usually contain the API blended with lactose as an excipient which acts [among other things] to provide stability to the formulation, improve the flowability of the powder during manufacturing, and as a bulking agent in powder uptake from the device during inhalation and aerosolization. Particles of the API stick to the larger carrier particles of lactose by physical forces of interaction and are separated from the carrier when the device is actuated and the powder is inhaled (17).

Lactose may contain milk proteins, and this is stated in the Description section of the Full Prescribing Information for DPI products containing lactose. The presence of milk proteins may be a potential safety issue for people with significant milk allergies. Following the initial approval of Advair Diskus (fluticasone propionate and salmeterol inhalation powder, GlaxoSmithKline, Research Triangle Park, NC) in 2000, there were post-marketing reports of hypersensitivity reactions following administration of Advair Diskus in patients with severe milk protein allergy and the Full Prescribing Information was subsequently updated with a Contraindication and a Warning about this safety issue (18). A case report of a severe hypersensitivity reaction in a child with milk protein allergy following the administration of Advair Diskus was published in 2014 in the Journal of Pediatric Pharmacology Therapeutics (19). This experience is not unique to Advair Diskus and similar Warning and Contraindication statements can be found in other lactose-containing DPI products e.g., ASMANEX® TWISTHAER® (mometasone furoate inhalation powder, Merck & Co., INC, Whitehouse Station, NJ 08889, US) (20).

DEVICE-RELATED MEDICATION ERRORS

Unlike pMDI devices in which the dose is metered when the patient activates the device and breathes in, DPIs are available as multidose metered devices (e.g., ASMANEX TWISTHALER), single-dose devices (e.g., SPIRIVA® Handihaler®), and multiple unit dose devices (e.g., BREO ELLIPTA) (see Chapter 6). SPIRIVA® Handihaler® is comprised of the inhalation device (the Handihaler®) and the formulation (i.e., tiotropium blended with lactose monohydrate) in single-dose capsules. In order to use the product, the patient must insert a single-dose capsule into the Handihaler with each use.

Following the approval of Spiriva® Handihaler® [in 2004], there were complaints regarding patients' mishandling of the capsules and mistakenly swallowing them rather than using them in the accompanying inhaler devices. Similar complaints with another single-dose DPI product [no longer marketed] Foradil® Aerolizer™ (formoterol fumarate inhalation powder, Novartis Pharmaceuticals Corporation, East Hanover, New Jersey) were reported. The FDA issued a public health advisory recommending that healthcare providers advise patients on the proper use of the capsules and that swallowing them was ineffective (21) and updated the label for SPIRIVA® HANDIHALER® with additional clarifying language and warnings that the capsules must not be swallowed (22).

COMBINATION PRODUCTS: DEVICE CONSIDERATIONS

Fixed-dose combination products of inhaled corticosteroids and long-acting beta-agonists (ICS/LABA), fixed-dose combinations of different classes of bronchodilators: long-acting anticholinergics, and long-acting beta-agonists (LAMA/LABA) and fixed-dose combination products of inhaled corticosteroids, long-acting anticholinergics, and long-acting beta-agonists (ICS/LAMA/LABA) have been approved in a number of different devices and formulations including pressurized metered dose inhalers, dry powder inhalers in various prototypes, and more recently, a slow mist inhaler platform. Fixed-dose combination products provide the convenience of having two or more medications that a patient would otherwise be taking in two separate inhalers combined in a single inhaler. These combinations have been considered an improvement in the therapeutic armamentarium for asthma and COPD because reducing the number of inhalers simplifies treatment regimens. Such simplification of medication administration for patients has been shown in clinical studies to improve patient compliance and reduce healthcare resource utilization (23, 24).

From a regulatory perspective, there must be assurance, however, that not only these combinations are safe and effective, but that they provide a benefit over the individual active ingredients. Thus, the development of these products must satisfy the regulatory requirement that each active ingredient in the combination makes a contribution to the claimed effects of the combination product and that the combination is safe and effective for a significant patient population requiring such concurrent therapy as defined in the labeling for the drug (25).

For these fixed-dose combination products, device considerations involve [among other things] that drug developers provide data showing a lack of pharmaceutical interaction of the individual ingredients within the device. Typically, such information would ordinarily be provided with data that demonstrate that there is pharmaceutical comparability between the single ingredients as delivered by the combination and the corresponding single-ingredient drug products. In general, this would be achieved using the same device for the monotherapy and combination drug products and using formulations for the monotherapy products that have qualitative and quantitative comparability to that used for the combination drug products. In addition, demonstrating that the *in vitro* dose delivery and aerodynamic particle size distribution for each of the individual active ingredients are comparable across the monotherapy and combination products are necessary to provide assurance that the dose of each ingredient delivered from the combination product is the same as the dose delivered from the single-ingredient products.

Using exactly the same device and formulation (except for active ingredients) significantly reduces the complexities in demonstrating comparability. However, device sameness may not always be achievable for comparability. Device and/or formulation differences between the comparators can complicate the development of these combination products because it makes the demonstration of comparability [while surmountable] more challenging. For example, with the development of DULERA® (mometasone furoate and formoterol fumarate dihydrate, Merck & Co., Inc., Whitehouse Station, NJ, US) inhalation aerosol an ICS/LABA pMDI propelled with HFA-227, the formoterol monotherapy used in the clinical trials was different from the formoterol in the combination product (Dulera) in that the formoterol monotherapy product used HFA-134a as the propellant, and had lactose in the formulation as an excipient. Additionally, the inhaler device for the formoterol monotherapy product had a different valve than the combination product. Comparability between the formoterol single monotherapy product and Dulera was able to be established through various *in vitro* evaluations of drug-delivery characteristics (26).

Lack of pharmaceutical comparability between the combination product and the monotherapy comparators presents additional complexities to the development of fixed-dose combination products. In the clinical studies for the development of Symbicort® (budesonide and formoterol dihydrate, AstraZeneca Pharmaceuticals LP, Wilmington, DE) inhalation aerosol, a pharmaceutically different formoterol monotherapy comparator was used in the clinical studies. Symbicort is an inhalation aerosol formulation propelled by HFA-227. However, the formoterol single-ingredient comparator used in the clinical trials was the Oxis Turbohaler (formoterol fumarate dihydrate, AstraZeneca, UK Limited) a dry powder formulation of formoterol. A pharmacodynamic approach comparing bronchodilatory effects of various doses of formoterol administered via the Oxis Turbohaler or from Symbicort on a constant background of a fixed dose of budesonide was used to ensure that the formoterol delivered either from the dry powder formulation (Oxis Turbohaler) or from the inhalation aerosol (Symbicort) produced comparable bronchodilation (27, 28).

Ensuring pharmaceutical comparability between single- and corresponding dual-combination products can have the advantage of streamlining the drug development program for combination products that contain more than two active ingredients. For example, with the initial approval of TRELEGY ELLIPTA (fluticasone furoate, umeclidinium, and vilanterol inhalation powder, GlaxoSmithKline, Research Triangle Park, NC, US) the FDA accepted the data generated from clinical trials completed with the dual-combination product, BREO ELLIPTA (fluticasone furoate and vilanterol inhalation powder, GlaxoSmithKline, Research Triangle Park, NC) and the single-ingredient product INCRUSE ELLIPTA (umeclidinium inhalation powder, GlaxoSmithKline, Research Triangle Park, NC, US) to support the efficacy of TRELEGY ELLIPTA to improve lung function in COPD. This streamlined approach to achieve approval of the triple-combination product was made possible because the product developers provided data to support the pharmaceutical sameness or comparability of the triple-combination product compared with the dual-combination products of the ICS/LABA (BREO ELLIPTA), the LAMA/LABA (ANORO ELLIPTA), and single-ingredient LAMA (INCRUSE ELLIPTA) and ICS (ARNUITY ELLIPTA) products (29).

The full prescribing information for TRELEGY ELLIPTA notes that "comparative *in vitro* data for drug delivery and aerodynamic particle size distribution of the delivered drugs fluticasone furoate, umeclidinium, and vilanterol demonstrated that there were no pharmaceutical interactions, and each drug was delivered in a comparable manner whether administered via a single ELLIPTA inhaler or from separate inhalers" (30).

DOSING CONSIDERATIONS

As is expected for all new products, establishing the appropriate dose and dosing regimen is of critical importance for orally inhaled products for asthma and COPD. The objective of dose-ranging studies is to select both an appropriate nominal dose and a dosing frequency that would ensure adequate efficacy and safety of the product for the proposed indication in that patient population. Less frequent dosing is one of the ways to simplify treatment regimens and potentially improve compliance with chronic dosing. As such, drug products with long-lasting efficacy that can be dosed once daily instead of multiple times per day are an attractive option for patients on chronic inhaler therapy. Establishing efficacy with once-daily dosing regimens, however, must be achieved without compromising safety or efficacy and dose exploration is always a critical part of this process. Once-daily dosing may not always provide better efficacy compared to a multiple-dose treatment regimen. Flovent Diskus (fluticasone propionate inhalation powder, GlaxoSmithKline) is an orally inhaled corticosteroid approved with a twice-daily dosing regimen. In clinical studies, efficacy for the same nominal dose administered as a once-daily dosing regimen compared to a twice-daily dosing regimen was numerically and statistically inferior to the same nominal dose given twice daily (31).

Sometimes, multiple clinical trials may be needed to select an appropriate nominal dose and dosing frequency that would provide an acceptable risk/benefit profile for the product. The development of TUDORZA™ PRESSAIR (aclidinium bromide inhalation powder, AstraZeneca Pharmaceuticals LP, Wilmington, DE) a long-acting anticholinergic bronchodilator, is an example of how these two elements of dosing (the nominal dose and dosing frequency) factor into determining efficacy and safety. Initial pivotal studies using a dose of 200 µg of aclidinium administered once daily showed that the trough FEV_1 (the primary endpoint) was statistically superior to placebo; however, the effect size was only 60 mL. The FDA raised concerns over the significance of this effect given its modest size compared to the FEV_1 response seen for other bronchodilators approved for COPD. The drug developer subsequently conducted additional dose exploration and pivotal studies using higher doses, and a twice-daily dosing regimen. A dose of 400 µg administered twice daily demonstrated acceptable bronchodilator efficacy and the product was approved at a dose of 400 µg administered twice daily (32).

When a new product contains an active moiety that had been previously approved for oral inhalation, dosing information from the approved product may be useful to help guide the initial dose selection for the new product. For example, with the development of Spiriva Respimat for COPD, the general clinical pharmacology and biopharmaceutics for tiotropium bromide had already been evaluated with the development of the SPIRIVA Handihaler product, and the appropriate dosing interval of once-daily dosing for tiotropium

Table 14.1: Comparative Pharmacokinetics: Spiriva Respimat vs. Spiriva Handihaler

	Spiriva Respimat 5 µg	Spiriva Respimat 10 µg	Spiriva Handihaler 18 µg
Study 249	26.1	64.6	20.2
AUC 0–6 ss, pg.h/mL	63.5	148	52.2
AUC 0–24 ss, pg.h/mL	561	1230	428
Urinary Excretion 0–12 h, ng			

Source: United States Food and Drug Administration. Application no. 021936 summary review (33).

Abbreviation: ss = steady state.

bromide for COPD had been established. Therefore, dosing considerations for the Respimat product were for selection of the nominal dose. An assessment of the systemic exposure of tiotropium delivered from Spiriva Respimat compared with the systemic exposure of tiotropium delivered from the previously approved Spiriva Handihaler product was a key safety consideration. Because these products are locally acting, pharmacokinetic comparisons provide support for the nominal dose selection from the perspective of systemic safety; however, dedicated clinical trials were conducted to establish efficacy and further evaluate safety.

As shown in Table 14.1, data from one of the pharmacokinetic studies demonstrate that the systemic exposure of tiotropium 5 µg from the Respimat is a closer match to the systemic exposure of tiotropium 18 µg from Spiriva Handihaler compared to tiotropium 10 µg from the Respimat. Pivotal clinical efficacy and safety trials supported the 5 µg dose (2 inhalations of 2.5 µg per spray once daily) for COPD which is the approved dose (33).

HUMAN FACTORS

Device considerations for orally inhaled products also include human factors testing. That is, the evaluation that the device itself will be safe and effective for the intended users, uses, and use environments (34). Depending on the complexity of the device, human factors testing may also include specific patient use studies. The FDA has published guidance on the type of human factors studies and related clinical study considerations that should be taken into account with respect to combination products (35). Dedicated patient use studies were conducted with the Respimat platform to evaluate the use of the device in patients' hands prior to approval. Currently, there are four bronchodilator Respimat products on the market: Combivent Respimat (ipratropium bromide and albuterol), Spiriva Respimat (tiotropium bromide), Striverdi Respimat (olodaterol hydrochloride), and Stiolto Respimat (olodaterol hydrochloride and tiotropium bromide). For the approval of the first Respimat product (Combivent), the manufacturer completed human factors testing and patient handling studies, so these studies did not need to be repeated for subsequent products. The Respimat inhaler is the same device for all the products, but the cartridge containing the medication in solution is different for each product. While the Respimat platform is quite complex (compared to other orally inhaled platforms), this innovation allows for several advantages from the patient's perspective. Once assembled, the product is easy to use as the need for breath coordination (as needed for pMDIs) is not a factor. However, it was noted in patient handling studies that initial assembly of the product (i.e., inserting the cartridge into the base of the inhaler) could be problematic for some older patients or patients with joint problems of the hand and assistance may be needed with initial assembly (33). The fine particle aerosol mist generated with this platform results in a higher fine particle size allowing for more product to deposit in the lower airways. Aerosol is generated from this propellant-free product when the base is turned 180 degrees and the release button is pressed. A metered volume of the solution is expressed through a nozzle creating a fine mist (36) (see Chapter 5).

DOSE COUNTING MECHANISMS

Dose counting mechanisms are an integral part of DPI devices; however, the same is not the case with pMDIs. Knowing when to replace a pMDI was a challenge until a dose-counting mechanism was incorporated into the device. Prior to this advancement, unreliable methods such as manually counting doses, and testing whether the inhaler would float in water were some of the measures used by consumers to decide when to replace their inhalers. Such unreliable methods were problematic both from a safety and efficacy standpoint particularly with respect to short-acting bronchodilator inhalers used for quick relief of acute symptoms of airflow obstruction (37). Since the publication of the FDA guidance on dose counters (38), all pMDIs are now developed with a counting mechanism so that patients can confidently know when it is time to replace their inhalers. This is particularly helpful for short-acting bronchodilator products that are not typically used on a regular daily basis.

PEDIATRIC CONSIDERATIONS

Orally inhaled asthma products for pediatric patients include all of the general considerations previously discussed for drug-device combination products as well as issues specifically related to pediatric patients. Since systemic drug exposure to orally inhaled products cannot predict efficacy or define all aspects of the safety of these products, clinical trials are needed to evaluate safety and efficacy in the pediatric population. In general, dedicated pediatric studies are conducted in patients under 12 years of age, whereas patients 12 years of age and older are included (with some exceptions) in adult asthma studies. Separate evaluations across various age ranges in these pediatric studies are necessary because it cannot be assumed that efficacy in one age range would translate to efficacy across all pediatric age ranges. For example, available data from some short-acting bronchodilator studies show a lack of efficacy in children less than 4 years of age. A clinical trial conducted with XOPENEX HFA (levalbuterol tartrate, Sunovion Pharmaceuticals Inc., Marlborough, MA) in children less than 4 years of age showed no statistically significant difference between XOPENEX HFA and placebo. There was also an increased incidence of asthma-related adverse reactions compared to placebo in that study (39). Clinical trials with Ventolin HFA (albuterol sulfate inhalation aerosol, GlaxoSmithKline, Research Triangle Park, NC) in children under 4 years of age did not establish efficacy (40). The full prescribing information for Proventil HFA (albuterol sulfate, Merck & Co., Inc.; Whitehouse Station, NJ, US) and PROAIR-HFA (albuterol sulfate, Teva Respiratory LLC, Frazer, PA, US) do not describe any studies conducted in children under 4 years of age and state that safety and efficacy in pediatric patients under 4 years of age have not been established (41, 42).

A concern with pMDIs and pediatric patients is inhaler technique, and spacer devices are often used to address this issue. *In vitro* characterization studies must be conducted with spacers to ensure adequate drug delivery when they are used with pMDIs because inhalation times and other factors may impact drug delivery. For instance, the use of QVAR® inhalation aerosol (beclomethasone dipropionate HFA, Teva Respiratory LLC, Frazer, PA, US) with a spacer in children less than 5 years of age is not recommended because *in vitro* studies showed that the amount of medication delivered through the spacer decreased rapidly with increasing wait times of 5–10 seconds. The QVAR label recommends that if QVAR is used with a spacer device it is important to inhale immediately (43).

CONCLUSIONS

Orally inhaled products are the cornerstone of the therapeutic management of asthma and COPD. These products are complex dosage forms, and both the drug formulation and device components can impact the safety and efficacy of these products. Both components (formulation and device) are fully evaluated during development and undergo extensive testing to assure safety and efficacy prior to being placed on the market. Consumers can be assured that approval of these products for marketing only occurs after satisfactory fulfillment of all regulatory requirements with adherence to the highest scientific standards.

Disclaimer: Dr. Gilbert-McClain serves as a regulatory consultant to the pharmaceutical industry providing clinical and regulatory advice regarding their drug development programs. Confidentiality agreements preclude naming these companies. Dr Gilbert-McClain worked at the Food and Drug Administration in the review division that regulates the development of drugs for asthma and COPD but does not represent the agency and all information discussed in this chapter is in the public domain and the opinions expressed are her own.

REFERENCES

1. Alangari AA. Corticosteroids in the treatment of acute asthma. Ann Thorac Med 2014;9(4):187–192.
2. Clark TJ. Effect of beclomethasone dipropionate delivered by aerosol in patients with asthma. Lancet 1972;1:1361–1364.
3. United States Food and Drug Administration. Vanceril. Application no. 017573. Approval. [cited 2022 Feb 15]. Available from: https://www.accessdata.fda.gov/scripts/cder/daf/index.cfm?event=overview.process&ApplNo=01753
4. Code of Federal Regulations 21 CFR §312 (IND regulations) and 21 CFR §314 (NDA regulations). https://www.ecfr.gov/current/title-21/chapter-I/subchapter-D
5. [cited 2022 Mar 23]. Available from: https://www.fda.gov/drugs/guidances-drugs/product-specific-guidances-generic-drug-development
6. Guidance for Industry: Metered Dose inhaler (MDI) and Dry Powder Inhaler (DPI) Drug Products. Chemistry, Manufacturing, and Controls Documentation. Draft Guidance. [cited 2022 Feb 16]. Available from: https://www.fda.gov/media/70851/download
7. United States Food and Drug Administration. Application no. 204275. Full prescribing information. [cited 2022 Mar 23]. Available from: https://www.accessdata.fda.gov/drugsatfda_docs/label/2019/204275s017lbl.pdf

8. United States Food and Drug Administration. Application no. 204275. CMC reviews.[cited 2022 Jan 20]. Available from: https://www.accessdata. foda.gov/drugsatfda_docs/nda/2013/204275Orig1s000ChemR.pdf accessed 1/20/2022 https://www.accessdata.fda.gov/drugsatfda_docs/ nda/2013/203975Orig1s000ChemR.pdf

9. United States Food and Drug Administration. Combivent® Respimat® Full Prescribing Information. [cited 2022 Jan 10]. Available from: https://www. accessdata.fda.gov/drugsatfda_docs/label/2011/021742000lbl.pdf

10. United States Food and Drug Administration. Application no. 021747. Summary Review. [cited 2022 Feb 20]. Available from: https://www. accessdata.fda.gov/drugsatfda_docs/nda/2011/021747Orig1s000SumR.pdf

11. United States Food and Drug Administration. Application no. 021747. FDA action letter. [cited 2022 Feb 23]. Available from: https://www. accessdata.fda.ogv/drugsatfda_docs/nda/2011/021747Orig1s000Other ActionLtrs.pdf

12. United States Food and Drug Administration. Application no. 021747. FDA Review: Administrative Documents (s) & Correspondence. [cited 2022 Feb 23]. Available from: https://www.accessdata.fda.gov/drugsatfda_docs/nda /2011/021747Orig1s000AdminCorres.pdf

13. Fiore K. Doctors hear gripes about HFA inhalers. MedPage Today. [updated 2009 Mar 11; cited 2022 Feb 23]. Available from: https://www. medpagetoday.com/allergyimmunology/asthma/13227

14. United States Food and Drug Administration. Frequently asked questions. Transition from CFC propelled albuterol inhalers to HFA albuterol inhalers: Questions and Answers. [cited 2022 Feb 23]. Available from: https://www.fda.gov/drugs/questions-answers/transition-cfc-propelled-albuterol-inhalers-hfa-propelled-albuterol-inhalers-questions-and-answers

15. United States Food and Drug Administration. Xopenex HFA. Full prescribing information. [cited 2022 Mar 23]. Available from: https://www. accessdata.fda.gov/drugatfda_dcos/label/2017/021730s039labl/pdf

16. Schroeder AC. Leachables and extractables in OINDP: An FDA perspective. Presented at the PQRI Leachables and extractables Workshop, Bethesda, Maryland, December 5–6, 2005. [cited 2022 Jan 12]. Available from: https://pqri.org/wp-content/uploads/2015/08/pdf/ AlanSchroederDay1.pdf

17. Pilcer G, Wauthoz N, Amighi K. Lactose characteristics and the generation of the aerosol. Adv Drug Deliv Rev 2012;64(3):233–256.

18. United States Food and Drug Administration. Full prescribing information Advair Diskus 2008. [cited 2022 Mar 24]. Available from: https://www. accessdata.foda.goc/drugsatfda_docs/label/2008/021077s029lbl.pdf

19. Robles J, Motheral L. Hypersensitivity reaction after inhalation of a lactose-containing dry powder inhaler. J Pediatr Pharmacol Ther 2014;19(3):206–211.

20. United States Food and Drug Administration. Full prescribing information for Asmanex Twisthaler. [cited 2022 Mar 24]. Available from: https://www. accesdata.fda.gov/drugsatfda_docs/label/2021/021067s032lbl.pdf

21. FDA warns on Mistaken Ingestion of Inhaled Spiriva and Foradil Capsules. Medical News. Physician's First Watch. NEJM Journal Watch. [cited 2008 Mar 3]. Available from: https://www.jwatch.org/fw200803030000001/2008/03/03/ fda-warns-mistaken-ingestion-inhaled-spiriva-and

22. United States Food and Drug Administration. Spiriva Handihaler. Approval letter 021395s033ltr. [cited 2022 Feb 2]. Available from: https://www.accessdata.fda.gov/drugsatfda_docs/appletter/2011/021395s033ltr.pdf

23. Yu AP, Guerin A, de Leon DP, et al. Clinical and economic outcomes of multiple versus single long-acting inhalers in COPD. Respir Med 2011;105(12):1861–1871. DOI:10.1016/j.rmed.2011.07.001

24. Marceau C, Lemiere C, Berbiche D, et al. Persistence, adherence, and effectiveness of combination therapy among adult patients with asthma. J Allergy Clin Immunol 2006;118(3):574–581. DOI:10.1016/j.jaci.2006.06.034

25. Code of Federal Regulations 21CFR 300.50. [cited 2022 Mar 25]. Available from: https://www.ecfr.gov/current/title-21/chapter-1/subchapter-D/part-300/subpart-B/section-300.50

26. United States Food and Drug Administration. Application no. 022518Orig1s000 summary review. [cited 2022 Mar 28]. Available from: https://www.accessdata.fda.gov/drugsatfda_docs/nda/2010/022518Orig1s000SumR.pdf

27. United States Food and Drug Administration. Application no. 021929 office director memo. [cited 2022 Mar 28]. Available from: https://www.accessdata.fda.gov/drugsatfda_docs/nda/2006/021929s000_ODMemo.pdf

28. Miller CJ, Senn S, Mezzanotte WS. Bronchodilation of formoterol administered with budesonide: Device and formulation effects. Contemp Clin Trials 2008;29(2):114–124.

29. United States Food and Drug Administration. Application no. 209482. Summary review. [cited 2022 Feb 2]. Available from: https://www.accessdata.fda.gov/drugsatfda_docs/nda/2017/209482Orig1s000SumR.pdf

30. United States Food and Drug Administration. Trelegy Ellipta. Full Prescribing information. [cited 2022 Mar 30]. Available from: https://accessdata.fda.gov/drugsatfda_docs/label/2017/209482s000lbl.pdf

31. Purucker ME, Rosebraugh CJ, Zhou F, et al. Inhaled fluticasone propionate by diskus in the treatment of asthma: A comparison of the efficacy of the same nominal dose given either once or twice daily. Chest 2003;124(4):1584–1593.

32. United States Food and Drug Administration. Application no. 202450. Summary review. [cited 2022 Mar 22]. Available from: https://www.accessdata.fda.gov/drugsatfda_docs/nda/2012/202450Orig1s000SumR.pdf

33. United States Food and Drug Administration. Application no. 021936. Summary review. [cited 2022 Mar 22]. Available from: https://www.accessdata.fda.gov/drugsatfda_docs/nda/2014/021936Orig1s000SumR.pdf

34. United States Food and Drug Administration. Guidance for industry and Food and Drug Administration Staff. Applying human factors and usability engineering to medical devices. [updated 2016 Feb; cited 2022 Mar 29]. Available from: https://www.fda.gov/media/80481/download

35. United States Food and Drug Administration. Draft Guidance for industry and FDA Staff. Human Factors Studies and Related Clinical Study Considerations in Combination Product Design and Development. [updated 2016 Feb; cited 2022 Mar 29]. Available from: https://www.fda.gov/media/96018/download

36. United States Food and Drug Administration. Application no. 021936. Response to Device Consult Request. Other Reviews. [cited 2022 Mar 29]. Available from: https://www.accessdata.fda.gov/drugsatfda_docs/nda/2014/021936Orig1s000OtherR.pdf

37. Sander N, Fusco-Walkert SJ, Harder JM, et al. Dose counting and the use of pressurized metered-dose inhalers: Running on empty. Ann Allergy Asthma Immunol 2006;97(1):34–38.
38. United States Food and Drug Administration. Guidance for industry. Integration of dose-counting mechanisms into MDI drug products. [cited 2003 Mar 2]. Available from: https://www.fda.gov/media/71073/download
39. United States Food and Drug Administration. Xopenex HFA. Full Prescribing Information. [cited 2022 Mar 30]. Available from: https://www.accessdata.fda.gov/drugsatfda_docs/label/2017/021730s039lbl.pdf
40. United States Food and Drug Administration. Ventolin HFA. Full Prescribing information. [cited 2022 Mar 30]. Available from: https://www.accessdata.fda.gov/drugsatfda_docs/label/2021/020983s041lbl.pdf
41. United States Food and Drug Administration. Proventil HFA. Full Prescribing information. [cited 2022 Mar 30]. Available from: https://www.accessdata.fda.gov/drugsatfda_docs/label/2017/020503s054lbl.pdf
42. United States Food and Drug Administration. ProAir HFA. Full Prescribing Information. [cited 2022 Mar 30]. Available from: https://www.accessdata.fda.gov/drugsatfda_docs/label/2019/021457s036lbl.pdf
43. United States Food and Drug Administration. QVAR inhalation aerosol. Full Prescribing information. [cited 2022 Mar 10]. Available from: https://www.accessdata.fda.gov/drugsatfda_docs/label/2017/020911s030lbl.pdf

Index

Note: Locators in *italics* represent figures and **bold** indicate tables in the text.

9781032215730